Cooperative Reference: Social Interaction in the Workplace

Cooperative Reference: Social Interaction in the Workplace has been co-published simultaneously as *The Reference Librarian*, Numbers 83/84 2003.

The Reference Librarian Monographic "Separates"

Below is a list of "separates," which in serials librarianship means a special issue simultaneously published as a special journal issue or double-issue *and* as a "separate" hardbound monograph. (This is a format which we also call a "DocuSerial.")

"Separates" are published because specialized libraries or professionals may wish to purchase a specific thematic issue by itself in a format which can be separately cataloged and shelved, as opposed to purchasing the journal on an on-going basis. Faculty members may also more easily consider a "separate" for classroom adoption.

"Separates" are carefully classified separately with the major book jobbers so that the journal tie-in can be noted on new book order slips to avoid duplicate purchasing.

You may wish to visit Haworth's Website at . . .

http://www.HaworthPress.com

. . . to search our online catalog for complete tables of contents of these separates and related publications.

You may also call 1-800-HAWORTH (outside US/Canada: 607-722-5857), or Fax 1-800-895-0582 (outside US/Canada: 607-771-0012), or e-mail at:

docdelivery@haworthpress.com

Cooperative Reference: Social Interaction in the Workplace, edited by Celia Hales Mabry, PhD (No. 83/84, 2003). *This informative volume focuses on effective social interactions between library co-workers, presenting perspectives, firsthand accounts, and advice from experienced and successful reference librarians.*

Outreach Services in Academic and Special Libraries, edited by Paul Kelsey, MLIS, and Sigrid Kelsey, MLIS (No. 82, 2003). *Presents an array of models and case studies for creating and implementing outreach services in academic and special library settings.*

Managing the Twenty-First Century Reference Department: Challenges and Prospects, edited by Kwasi Sarkodie-Mensah, PhD (No. 81, 2003). *An up-to-date guide on managing and maintaining a reference department in the twenty-first century.*

Digital Reference Services, edited by Bill Katz, PhD (No. 79/80, 2002/2003). *A clear and concise book explaining developments in electronic technology for reference services and their implications for reference librarians.*

The Image and Role of the Librarian, edited by Wendi Arant, MLS, and Candace R. Benefiel, MA, MLIS (No. 78, 2002). *A unique and insightful examination of how librarians are perceived–and how they perceive themselves.*

Distance Learning: Information Access and Services for Virtual Users, edited by Hemalata Iyer, PhD (No. 77, 2002). *Addresses the challenge of providing Web-based library instructional materials in a time of ever-changing technologies.*

Helping the Difficult Library Patron: New Approaches to Examining and Resolving a Long-Standing and Ongoing Problem, edited by Kwasi Sarkodie-Mensah, PhD (No. 75/76, 2002). *"Finally! A book that fills in the information cracks not covered in library school about the ubiquitous problem patron. Required reading for public service librarians." (Cheryl LaGuardia, MLS, Head of Instructional Services for the Harvard College Library, Cambridge, Massachusetts)*

Evolution in Reference and Information Services: The Impact of the Internet, edited by Di Su, MLS (No. 74, 2001). *Helps you make the most of the changes brought to the profession by the Internet.*

Doing the Work of Reference: Practical Tips for Excelling as a Reference Librarian, edited by Celia Hales Mabry, PhD (No. 72 and 73, 2001). *"An excellent handbook for reference librarians who wish to move from novice to expert. Topical coverage is extensive and is presented by the best guides possible: practicing reference librarians." (Rebecca Watson-Boone, PhD, President, Center for the Study of Information Professionals, Inc.)*

Celia Hales Mabry
Editor

Cooperative Reference: Social Interaction in the Workplace

Cooperative Reference: Social Interaction in the Workplace has been co-published simultaneously as *The Reference Librarian*, Numbers 83/84 2003.

Pre-publication REVIEWS, COMMENTARIES, EVALUATIONS . . .

"**N**o reference librarian is an island, entire of herself. The complementary chapters Celia Mabry has commissioned and brought together explore the interconnectedness and interdependence of colleagues in a single reference department, of reference librarians and those whom they serve, of the reference department and the rest of the library, of the virtual and the traditional library, and of any library and other libraries. The authors emphasize practice and practitioners. THOSE LOOKING FOR IDEAS TO IMPROVE SERVICE OR SEEKING A DEEPER UNDERSTANDING OF THE 'WHYS' UNDERPINNING PRACTICE WILL FIND MUCH OF VALUE. Cooperation tells only part of the story. This book shows that collaboration–a deeper, more engaged form of interaction than co-operation–pervades contemporary reference service and gives it a strength that no insular approach could achieve."

James Rettig, MALS, MA
University Librarian
Boatwright Memorial Library
University of Richmond

More pre-publication
REVIEWS, COMMENTARIES, EVALUATIONS . . .

"There are some EXCELLENT CASE STUDIES in this comprehensive treatment of cooperative reference work in academic libraries. Celia Hayes Mabry establishes a remarkably forthright tone in her introduction. Joseph E. Straw gives the topic a valuable historical context in his conclusion to the volume. In between are A NUMBER OF INTERESTING EXAMPLES OF PROFESSIONALS WORKING IN COOPERATION WITH EACH OTHER, WITH STUDENTS, AND WITH FACULTY. . . . Millet's and Lister's chapters offer solid introductions to the basics of 'library culture' and how successful and collegial work actually occurs. . . . Other chapters, such as the Hull and Taylor contribution on P-16 educational support, amply illustrate collaboration between LIS professionals across workplaces. My favorite is King's explication of reference desk scheduling. ANYONE WHO HAS EITHER HAD TO DEVELOP OR ABIDE BY A SCHEDULE WILL WANT TO READ THIS! The system used is clearly and completely described, and the benefits seen in the cooperation between reference staff members underscores the focus of this entire book."

Rebecca Watson-Boone, PhD
Independent Scholar/Researcher

"A MUST for every new and seasoned librarian interested in the social character of reference service; a practical collection of the how and why of cooperation and collaboration."

JoAnn DeVries, MLS
Associate Librarian
University of Minnesota Libraries

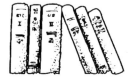

New Technologies and Reference Services, edited by Bill Katz, PhD (No. 71, 2000). *This important book explores developing trends in publishing, information literacy in the reference environment, reference provision in adult basic and community education, searching sessions, outreach programs, locating moving image materials for multimedia development, and much more.*

Reference Services for the Adult Learner: Challenging Issues for the Traditional and Technological Era, edited by Kwasi Sarkodie-Mensah, PhD (No. 69/70, 2000). *Containing research from librarians and adult learners from the United States, Canada, and Australia, this comprehensive guide offers you strategies for teaching adult patrons that will enable them to properly use and easily locate all of the materials in your library.*

Library Outreach, Partnerships, and Distance Education: Reference Librarians at the Gateway, edited by Wendi Arant and Pixey Anne Mosley (No. 67/68, 1999). *Focuses on community outreach in libraries toward a broader public by extending services based on recent developments in information technology.*

From Past-Present to Future-Perfect: A Tribute to Charles A. Bunge and the Challenges of Contemporary Reference Service, edited by Chris D. Ferguson, PhD (No. 66, 1999). *Explore reprints of selected articles by Charles Bunge, bibliographies of his published work, and original articles that draw on Bunge's values and ideas in assessing the present and shaping the future of reference service.*

Reference Services and Media, edited by Martha Merrill, PhD (No. 65, 1999). *Gives you valuable information about various aspects of reference services and media, including changes, planning issues, and the use and impact of new technologies.*

Coming of Age in Reference Services: A Case History of the Washington State University Libraries, edited by Christy Zlatos, MSLS (No. 64, 1999). *A celebration of the perseverance, ingenuity, and talent of the librarians who have served, past and present, at the Holland Library reference desk.*

Document Delivery Services: Contrasting Views, edited by Robin Kinder, MLS (No. 63, 1999). *Reviews the planning and process of implementing document delivery in four university libraries–Miami University, University of Colorado at Denver, University of Montana at Missoula, and Purdue University Libraries.*

The Holocaust: Memories, Research, Reference, edited by Robert Hauptman, PhD, and Susan Hubbs Motin (No. 61/62, 1998). *"A wonderful resource for reference librarians, students, and teachers . . . on how to present this painful, historical event." (Ephraim Kaye, PhD, The International School for Holocaust Studies, Yad Vashem, Jerusalem)*

Electronic Resources: Use and User Behavior, edited by Hemalata Iyer, PhD (No. 60, 1998). *Covers electronic resources and their use in libraries, with emphasis on the Internet and the Geographic Information Systems (GIS).*

Philosophies of Reference Service, edited by Celia Hales Mabry (No. 59, 1997). *"Recommended reading for any manager responsible for managing reference services and hiring reference librarians in any type of library." (Charles R. Anderson, MLS, Associate Director for Public Services, King County Library System, Bellevue, Washington)*

Business Reference Services and Sources: How End Users and Librarians Work Together, edited by Katherine M. Shelfer (No. 58, 1997). *"This is an important collection of papers suitable for all business librarians. . . . Highly recommended!" (Lucy Heckman, MLS, MBA, Business and Economics Reference Librarian, St. John's University, Jamaica, New York)*

Reference Sources on the Internet: Off the Shelf and onto the Web, edited by Karen R. Diaz (No. 57, 1997). *Surf off the library shelves and onto the Internet and cut your research time in half!*

Reference Services for Archives and Manuscripts, edited by Laura B. Cohen (No. 56, 1997). *"Features stimulating and interesting essays on security in archives, ethics in the archival profession, and electronic records." ("The Year's Best Professional Reading" (1998), Library Journal)*

Career Planning and Job Searching in the Information Age, edited by Elizabeth A. Lorenzen, MLS (No. 55, 1996). *"Offers stimulating background for dealing with the issues of technology and service. . . . A reference tool to be looked at often." (The One-Person Library)*

The Roles of Reference Librarians: Today and Tomorrow, edited by Kathleen Low, MLS (No. 54, 1996). *"A great asset to all reference collections. . . . Presents important, valuable information for reference librarians as well as other library users." (Library Times International)*

Reference Services for the Unserved, edited by Fay Zipkowitz. MSLS, DA (No. 53, 1996). *"A useful tool in developing strategies to provide services to all patrons."* (Science Books & Films)

Library Instruction Revisited: Bibliographic Instruction Comes of Age, edited by Lyn Elizabeth M. Martin, MLS (No. 51/52, 1995). *"A powerful collection authored by respected practitioners who have stormed the bibliographic instruction (BI) trenches and, luckily for us, have recounted their successes and shortcomings."* (The Journal of Academic Librarianship)

Library Users and Reference Services, edited by Jo Bell Whitlatch, PhD (No. 49/50, 1995). *"Well-planned, balanced, and informative. . . . Both new and seasoned professionals will find material for service attitude formation and practical advice for the front lines of service."* (Anna M. Donnelly, MS, MA, Associate Professor and Reference Librarian, St. John's University Library)

Social Science Reference Services, edited by Pam Baxter, MLS (No. 48, 1995). *"Offers practical guidance to the reference librarian. . . . A valuable source of information about specific literatures within the social sciences and the skills and techniques needed to provide access to those literatures."* (Nancy P. O'Brien, MLS, Head, Education and Social Science Library, and Professor of Library Administration, University of Illinois at Urbana-Champaign)

Reference Services in the Humanities, edited by Judy Reynolds, MLS (No. 47, 1994). *"A well-chosen collection of situations and challenges encountered by reference librarians in the humanities."* (College Research Library News)

Racial and Ethnic Diversity in Academic Libraries: Multicultural Issues, edited by Deborah A. Curry, MLS, MA, Susan Griswold Blandy, MEd, and Lyn Elizabeth M. Martin, MLS (No. 45/46, 1994). *"The useful techniques and attractive strategies presented here will provide the incentive for fellow professionals in academic libraries around the country to go and do likewise in their own institutions."* (David Cohen, Adjunct Professor of Library Science, School of Library and Information Science, Queens College; Director, EMIE (Ethnic Materials Information Exchange); Editor, EMIE Bulletin)

School Library Reference Services in the 90s: Where We Are, Where We're Heading, edited by Carol Truett, PhD (No. 44, 1994). *"Unique and valuable to the the teacher-librarian as well as students of librarianship. . . . The overall work successfully interweaves the concept of the continuously changing role of the teacher-librarian."* (Emergency Librarian)

Reference Services Planning in the 90s, edited by Gail Z. Eckwright, MLS, and Lori M. Keenan, MLS (No. 43, 1994). *"This monograph is well-researched and definitive, encompassing reference service as practices by library and information scientists. . . . It should be required reading for all professional librarian trainees."* (Feliciter)

Librarians on the Internet: Impact on Reference Services, edited by Robin Kinder, MLS (No. 41/42, 1994). *"Succeeds in demonstrating that the Internet is becoming increasingly a challenging but practical and manageable tool in the reference librarian's ever-expanding armory."* (Reference Reviews)

Reference Service Expertise, edited by Bill Katz (No. 40, 1993). *This important volume presents a wealth of practical ideas for improving the art of reference librarianship.*

Modern Library Technology and Reference Services, edited by Samuel T. Huang, MLS, MS (No. 39, 1993). *"This book packs a surprising amount of information into a relatively few number of pages. . . . This book will answer many questions."* (Science Books and Films)

Assessment and Accountability in Reference Work, edited by Susan Griswold Blandy, Lyn M. Martin, and Mary L. Strife (No. 38, 1992). *"An important collection of well-written, real-world chapters addressing the central questions that surround performance and services in all libraries."* (Library Times International)

The Reference Librarian and Implications of Mediation, edited by M. Keith Ewing, MLS, and Robert Hauptman, MLS (No. 37, 1992). *"An excellent and thorough analysis of reference mediation. . . . Well worth reading by anyone involved in the delivery of reference services."* (Fred Batt, MLS, Associate University Librarian for Public Services, California State University, Sacramento)

Library Services for Career Planning, Job Searching and Employment Opportunities, edited by Byron Anderson, MA, MLS (No. 36, 1992). *"An interesting book which tells professional libraries how to set up career information centers. . . . Clearly valuable reading for anyone establishing a career library."* (Career Opportunities News)

In the Spirit of 1992: Access to Western European Libraries and Literature, edited by Mary M. Huston, PhD, and Maureen Pastine, MLS (No. 35, 1992). *"A valuable and practical [collection] which every subject specialist in the field would do well to consult." (Western European Specialists Section Newsletter)*

Access Services: The Convergence of Reference and Technical Services, edited by Gillian M. McCombs, ALA (No. 34, 1992). *"Deserves a wide readership among both technical and public services librarians. . . . Highly recommended for any librarian interested in how reference and technical services roles may be combined." (Library Resources & Technical Services)*

Opportunities for Reference Services: The Bright Side of Reference Services in the 1990s, edited by Bill Katz (No. 33, 1991). *"A well-deserved look at the brighter side of reference services. . . . Should be read by reference librarians and their administrators in all types of libraries." (Library Times International)*

Government Documents and Reference Services, edited by Robin Kinder, MLS (No. 32, 1991). *Discusses access possibilities and policies with regard to government information, covering such important topics as new and impending legislation, information on most frequently used and requested sources, and grant writing.*

The Reference Library User: Problems and Solutions, edited by Bill Katz (No. 31, 1991). *"Valuable information and tangible suggestions that will help us as a profession look critically at our users and decide how they are best served." (Information Technology and Libraries)*

Continuing Education of Reference Librarians, edited by Bill Katz (No. 30/31, 1990). *"Has something for everyone interested in this field. . . . Library trainers and library school teachers may well find stimulus in some of the programs outlined here." (Library Association Record)*

Weeding and Maintenance of Reference Collections, edited by Sydney J. Pierce, PhD, MLS (No. 29, 1990). *"This volume may spur you on to planned activity before lack of space dictates 'ad hoc' solutions." (New Library World)*

Serials and Reference Services, edited by Robin Kinder, MLS, and Bill Katz (No. 27/28, 1990). *"The concerns and problems discussed are those of serials and reference librarians everywhere. . . . The writing is of a high standard and the book is useful and entertaining. . . . This book can be recommended." (Library Association Record)*

Rothstein on Reference: . . . with some help from friends, edited by Bill Katz and Charles Bunge, PhD, MLS (No. 25/26, 1990). *"An important and stimulating collection of essays on reference librarianship. . . . Highly recommended!" (Richard W. Grefrath, MA, MLS, Reference Librarian, University of Nevada Library)* Dedicated to the work of Sam Rothstein, one of the world's most respected teachers of reference librarians, this special volume features his writings as well as articles written about him and his teachings by other professionals in the field.

Integrating Library Use Skills Into the General Education Curriculum, edited by Maureen Pastine, MLS, and Bill Katz (No. 24, 1989). *"All contributions are written and presented to a high standard with excellent references at the end of each. . . . One of the best summaries I have seen on this topic." (Australian Library Review)*

Expert Systems in Reference Services, edited by Christine Roysdon, MLS, and Howard D. White, PhD, MLS (No. 23, 1989). *"The single most comprehensive work on the subject of expert systems in reference service." (Information Processing and Management)*

Information Brokers and Reference Services, edited by Bill Katz and Robin Kinder, MLS (No. 22, 1989). *"An excellent tool for reference librarians and indispensable for anyone seriously considering their own information-brokering service." (Booklist)*

Information and Referral in Reference Services, edited by Marcia Stucklen Middleton, MLS, and Bill Katz (No. 21, 1988). *Investigates a wide variety of situations and models which fall under the umbrella of information and referral.*

Reference Services and Public Policy, edited by Richard Irving, MLS, and Bill Katz (No. 20, 1988). *Looks at the relationship between public policy and information and reports ways in which libraries respond to the need for public policy information.*

Finance, Budget, and Management for Reference Services, edited by Ruth A. Fraley, MLS, MBA, and Bill Katz (No. 19, 1989). *"Interesting and relevant to the current state of financial needs in reference service. . . . A must for anyone new to or already working in the reference service area." (Riverina Library Review)*

Current Trends in Information: Research and Theory, edited by Bill Katz and Robin Kinder, MLS (No. 18, 1987). *"Practical direction to improve reference services and does so in a variety of ways ranging from humorous and clever metaphoric comparisons to systematic and practical methodological descriptions." (American Reference Books Annual)*

International Aspects of Reference and Information Services, edited by Bill Katz and Ruth A. Fraley, MLS, MBA (No. 17, 1987). *"An informative collection of essays written by eminent librarians, library school staff, and others concerned with the international aspects of information work." (Library Association Record)*

Reference Services Today: From Interview to Burnout, edited by Bill Katz and Ruth A. Fraley, MLS, MBA (No. 16, 1987). *Authorities present important advice to all reference librarians on the improvement of service and the enhancement of the public image of reference services.*

The Publishing and Review of Reference Sources, edited by Bill Katz and Robin Kinder, MLS (No. 15, 1987). *"A good review of current reference reviewing and publishing trends in the United States . . . will be of interest to intending reviewers, reference librarians, and students." (Australasian College Libraries)*

Personnel Issues in Reference Services, edited by Bill Katz and Ruth Fraley, MLS, MBA (No. 14, 1986). *"Chock-full of information that can be applied to most reference settings. Recommended for libraries with active reference departments." (RQ)*

Reference Services in Archives, edited by Lucille Whalen (No. 13, 1986). *"Valuable for the insights it provides on the reference process in archives and as a source of information on the different ways of carrying out that process." (Library and Information Science Annual)*

Conflicts in Reference Services, edited by Bill Katz and Ruth A. Fraley, MLS, MBA (No. 12, 1985). *This collection examines issues pertinent to the reference department.*

Evaluation of Reference Services, edited by Bill Katz and Ruth A. Fraley, MLS, MBA (No. 11, 1985). *"A much-needed overview of the present state of the art vis-à-vis reference service evaluation. . . . Excellent. . . . Will appeal to reference professionals and aspiring students." (RQ)*

Library Instruction and Reference Services, edited by Bill Katz and Ruth A. Fraley, MLS, MBA (No. 10, 1984). *"Well written, clear, and exciting to read. This is an important work recommended for all librarians, particularly those involved in, interested in, or considering bibliographic instruction. . . . A milestone in library literature." (RQ)*

Reference Services and Technical Services: Interactions in Library Practice, edited by Gordon Stevenson and Sally Stevenson (No. 9, 1984). *"New ideas and longstanding problems are handled with humor and sensitivity as practical suggestions and new perspectives are suggested by the authors." (Information Retrieval & Library Automation)*

Reference Services for Children and Young Adults, edited by Bill Katz and Ruth A. Fraley, MLS, MBA (No. 7/8, 1983). *"Offers a well-balanced approach to reference service for children and young adults." (RQ)*

Video to Online: Reference Services in the New Technology, edited by Bill Katz and Ruth A. Fraley, MLS, MBA (No. 5/6, 1983). *"A good reference manual to have on hand. . . . Well-written, concise, provide[s] a wealth of information." (Online)*

Ethics and Reference Services, edited by Bill Katz and Ruth A. Fraley, MLS, MBA (No. 4, 1982). *Library experts discuss the major ethical and legal implications that reference librarians must take into consideration when handling sensitive inquiries about confidential material.*

Reference Services Administration and Management, edited by Bill Katz and Ruth A. Fraley, MLS, MBA (No. 3, 1982). *Librarianship experts discuss the management of the reference function in libraries and information centers, outlining the responsibilities and qualifications of reference heads.*

Reference Services in the 1980s, edited by Bill Katz (No. 1/2, 1982). *Here is a thought-provoking volume on the future of reference services in libraries, with an emphasis on the challenges and needs that have come about as a result of automation.*

Cooperative Reference: Social Interaction in the Workplace

Celia Hales Mabry
Editor

Cooperative Reference: Social Interaction in the Workplace has been co-published simultaneously as *The Reference Librarian*, Numbers 83/84 2003.

The Haworth Information Press®
An Imprint of The Haworth Press, Inc.

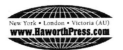

New York • London • Victoria (AU)
www.HaworthPress.com

Published by

The Haworth Information Press®, 10 Alice Street, Binghamton, NY 13904-1580 USA

The Haworth Information Press® is an imprint of The Haworth Press, Inc., 10 Alice Street, Binghamton, NY 13904-1580 USA.

Cooperative Reference: Social Interaction in the Workplace has been co-published simultaneously as *The Reference Librarian*™, Numbers 83/84 2003.

The development, preparation, and publication of this work has been undertaken with great care. However, the publisher, employees, editors, and agents of The Haworth Press and all imprints of The Haworth Press, Inc., including The Haworth Medical Press® and Pharmaceutical Products Press®, are not responsible for any errors contained herein or for consequences that may ensue from use of materials or information contained in this work. Opinions expressed by the author(s) are not necessarily those of The Haworth Press, Inc. With regard to case studies, identities and circumstances of individuals discussed herein have been changed to protect confidentiality. Any resemblance to actual persons, living or dead, is entirely coincidental.

Cover design by Lora Wiggins.

Library of Congress Cataloging-in-Publication Data

Cooperative reference : social interaction in the workplace / Celia Hales Mabry, editor.
    p. cm.
    "Co-published simultaneously as The reference librarian, numbers 83/84, 2003."
    Includes bibliographical references and index.
    ISBN 0-7890-2370-9 (alk. paper) – ISBN 0-7890-2371-7 (pbk. : alk. paper)
    1. Reference services (Libraries) 2. Electronic reference services (Libraries) 3. Reference librarians–Professional relationships. 4. Teams in the workplace. 5. Academic libraries–Reference services. 6. Reference services (Libraries)–United States. I. Hales-Mabry, Celia. II. Reference librarian.
Z711.C66 2003
025.5'2–dc22
                                                                                    2003024348

Indexing, Abstracting & Website/Internet Coverage

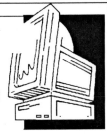

This section provides you with a list of major indexing & abstracting services. That is to say, each service began covering this periodical during the year noted in the right column. Most Websites which are listed below have indicated that they will either post, disseminate, compile, archive, cite or alert their own Website users with research-based content from this work. (This list is as current as the copyright date of this publication.)

(continued)

*Exact start date to come.

(continued)

*Special bibliographic notes related to special journal issues
(separates) and indexing/abstracting:*

- indexing/abstracting services in this list will also cover material in any "separate" that is co-published simultaneously with Haworth's special thematic journal issue or DocuSerial. Indexing/abstracting usually covers material at the article/chapter level.
- monographic co-editions are intended for either non-subscribers or libraries which intend to purchase a second copy for their circulating collections.
- monographic co-editions are reported to all jobbers/wholesalers/approval plans. The source journal is listed as the "series" to assist the prevention of duplicate purchasing in the same manner utilized for books-in-series.
- to facilitate user/access services all indexing/abstracting services are encouraged to utilize the co-indexing entry note indicated at the bottom of the first page of each article/chapter/contribution.
- this is intended to assist a library user of any reference tool (whether print, electronic, online, or CD-ROM) to locate the monographic version if the library has purchased this version but not a subscription to the source journal.
- individual articles/chapters in any Haworth publication are also available through the Haworth Document Delivery Service (HDDS).

Cooperative Reference:
Social Interaction in the Workplace

CONTENTS

ABOUT THE EDITOR

Celia Hales Mabry, PhD, is Reference Librarian and Bibliographer at the University of Minnesota's Wilson Library in Minneapolis, where she has worked since 1986. Dr. Mabry edited *Doing the Work of Reference: Practical Tips for Excelling as a Reference Librarian* (The Haworth Press, Inc., 2001) and *Philosophies of Reference Service* (The Haworth, Press, Inc., 1997); and authored *The World of the Aging: Information Needs and Choices* (American Library Association, 1993). She has the PhD from The Florida State University; the MLS from East Carolina University; and the BA and MA from Duke University.

Dr. Mabry lives in St. Paul with her husband, Paul D. Mabry, a neuroscientist on the faculty of the University of St. Thomas.

Introduction

Celia Hales Mabry

This subject of cooperation in the reference setting is quite close to my heart. I now have 20 years experience as a reference librarian, but it was not always so, and I had to learn, like everybody else, *how* to cooperate. When I began work as a reference librarian/English bibliographer at the University of North Carolina at Charlotte in 1983, I was not prepared to understand that virtually everything that I did impacted everyone else. My previous major experience had been as an instructor of freshman composition in a woman's college before the days of team-teaching and cooperative learning; in the classroom there were only the students and I, and if I didn't find something creative to do with them, it didn't get done.

Reference work and bibliographic instruction (as it was called then) demanded a different kind of work. It might have lacked the creativity that teaching allowed, but it more than made up for this lack by the tremendous opportunities for social interaction and working together on a team for a common purpose. My 17 years at the University of Minnesota Libraries have only amplified the tremendous benefits that we gain by working together. I now personally believe with great conviction that two heads are better than one–that the group consensus is going to be better than the thinking, however original, of only one individual.

The articles in this monograph are written from the firsthand experience of on-the-job reference librarians, and the cooperation that they expound upon is based on their grassroots experience. There is a place to explore cooperation more globally, but this publication is not the

[Haworth co-indexing entry note]: "Introduction." Mabry, Celia Hales. Co-published simultaneously in *The Reference Librarian* (The Haworth Information Press, an imprint of The Haworth Press, Inc.) No. 83/84, 2003, pp. 1-3; and: *Cooperative Reference: Social Interaction in the Workplace* (ed: Celia Hales Mabry) The Haworth Information Press, an imprint of The Haworth Press, Inc., 2003, pp. 1-3. Single or multiple copies of this article are available for a fee from The Haworth Document Delivery Service [1-800-HAWORTH, 9:00 a.m. - 5:00 p.m. (EST). E-mail address: docdelivery@haworthpress.com].

Digital Object Identifier: 10.1300J120v40n83_01   *1* place. This publication will give you as a reference librarian or administrator ideas to support cooperative efforts in the library's physical setting and then beyond the library walls, with the reference librarian doing the work.

The first section, "Serving at the Reference Desk," shows us in our most familiar milieu. The first three articles, by Pamela J. McKenzie, Michelle S. Millet, and Lisa F. Lister, point out ways to work together as reference librarians to improve our skills and service. In these three articles, we are working together. The fourth article in this section was contributed by this editor, Celia Hales Mabry, and it reaches across the reference desk to see our user on the other side as a partner in the reference transaction.

The next two sections complement each other as a pair: "Working Within the Library: Intangibles" and "Working Within the Library: Practicalities." The "intangibles" are explored by Lorraine J. Pellack, Corinne Laverty, and Melody Burton, and they point to those qualities of mind and heart that inform our working life, but with a cooperative spirit. The "practicalities" are explored by Tracy L. Hull, Natalia Taylor, Valery King, Della H. Darby, Lori A. Northrup, Carla T. Waddell, Heather F. Watters, Maria Anna Jankowska, Linnea Marshall, Teresa U. Berry, and Flora G. Shrode. These articles are filled with tips for improving our service to our users while we work within the walls of the physical library. We have not moved so far yet as to leave behind physical structure.

The fourth section can be seen as a preview of what lies ahead for reference service, "The Virtual Library: Outreach to Users." Here Debra Engel, Sarah Robbins, Eve M. Diel, Theresa K. Flett, Sharon Ladenson, Sherry Hawkins Backhus, Terri Pedersen Summey, Connie Ury, and Carolyn Johnson take a look at the library of the future as it is showing up now—websites, online tutorials, e-mail reference, distance education, and a more general overview of reference beyond the physical walls that also touches on faculty users.

"Cooperating with Faculty" comes next in line, as James Cory Tucker, Jeremy Bullian, Matthew C. Torrence, and Barbara J. D'Angelo reach beyond their companion reference librarians to cooperate within their larger community.

Finally, "Cooperating with Other Libraries" is explored by Karen A. Buxton, Harvey R. Gover, and Joseph E. Straw. The first of the two articles describes the challenges of combining two very different libraries at one service point; and the second is a sweeping assessment of library cooperation from the historical perspective, 1876 to 2002. This final article invites speculation of what the future will bring by grounding us in where we have been. We are now writing the sequel to what Joseph Straw details for us.

I would like to close with personal words. I work at the reference desk on the first floor of Wilson Library, University of Minnesota, Minneapolis, with individuals whom I have come to know and love over what is now a very long time. As I write this on May 15, 2003, they are as follows: Priscilla Angenor, Laura Dale Bischof, Tammy Bobrowsky, Kim Clarke, Bill Fietzer, Susan Gangl, Julianne Haahr, Laurel Haycock, Becky Hoffmann, Melissa Kalpin, Kay Kane, Barbara Kautz, Julia Kiple, Eugene Leadon, Dennis Lien, Kate McCready, Carla Pfahl, Gwen Schagrin, Lynn Skupeko, Kayellen Taylor, Jerilyn Veldof, and Mary Pat Winters. They provide the backdrop for my publishing activities, and they are supportive. So are our administrators, and I wish to thank specifically Kay Kane, our academic program director for the humanities and social sciences. I also cooperate with selectors and bibliographers in the humanities and social sciences whom I won't name here (you know who you are); their friendships are invaluable to me in my collections work, an adjunct to the reference service. All of us in our work world at the University of Minnesota Libraries are drawn as one cooperative body by the imaginative leadership of our University Librarian, Wendy Pradt Lougee.

I appreciate the e-mail mentorship that Bill Katz, our series editor for *The Reference Librarian*, has established with me. He is someone to emulate, someone who has kept involved in the profession at dizzying heights for a long time, but who is still most human in his interactions and his support. He deserves the tribute of reference librarians everywhere. The profession of reference librarianship would be in a very different place but for his lifelong contributions.

My husband, Paul Mabry, is a constant source of amazement to me. He is a very wise man who doesn't need to read the spiritual books that draw me ever more deeply into what it means to cooperate in this life. He lives these higher ideals as my romantic and day-to-day soulmate, and I thank him for always sharing and listening with keen insight and a warm heart.

User Perspectives
on Staff Cooperation
During the Reference Transaction

Pamela J. McKenzie

SUMMARY. Discussions of the reference transaction generally assume one staff member and one patron, but this is not always the case in practice. This paper reports on data collected from users' descriptions of public and academic library reference transactions in which more than one staff member played a part. It analyzes users' evaluations of effective and ineffective staff behavior in three aspects of the reference transaction: the initiation of the reference encounter, collaboration between staff members, and serial encounters with more than one staff member. It suggests some ways that guidelines for reference desk behavior might be extended to accommodate multi-staff transactions. *[Article copies available for a fee from The Haworth Document Delivery Service: 1-800-HAWORTH. E-mail address: <docdelivery@haworthpress.com> Website: <http://www.HaworthPress.com> © 2003 by The Haworth Press, Inc. All rights reserved.]*

Pamela J. McKenzie is Assistant Professor, Graduate Program, Library Information Science, Faculty of Information and Media Studies, The University of Western Ontario, London, Ontario, Canada N6A 5B7 (E-mail: pmckenzi@uwo.ca).

The author wishes to thank Catherine Ross and Kirsti Nilsen for their assistance and encouragement.

[Haworth co-indexing entry note]: "User Perspectives on Staff Cooperation During the Reference Transaction." McKenzie, Pamela J. Co-published simultaneously in *The Reference Librarian* (The Haworth Information Press, an imprint of The Haworth Press, Inc.) No. 83/84, 2003, pp. 5-22; and: *Cooperative Reference: Social Interaction in the Workplace* (ed: Celia Hales Mabry) The Haworth Information Press, an imprint of The Haworth Press, Inc., 2003, pp. 5-22. Single or multiple copies of this article are available for a fee from The Haworth Document Delivery Service [1-800-HAWORTH, 9:00 a.m. - 5:00 p.m. (EST). E-mail address: docdelivery@haworthpress.com].

Digital Object Identifier: 10.1300J120v40n83_02

KEYWORDS. Reference, user satisfaction, cooperation, collaboration, evaluation

INTRODUCTION

The literature on cooperation and collaboration in reference service often focuses on institutional-level cooperation, e.g., between institutions and groups of users (*Reference Services Review*, 2001); between or among libraries (Hogan, 1996); or between libraries and other agencies such as schools (Kahn, 2000). At the level of the librarian-patron interaction, however, there is little emphasis on cooperation. Writing about the reference transaction and guidelines for reference service generally assume one staff member and one patron. Very little has been written about what might happen when more than two people are involved in a reference transaction.

Chelton (1999) observed that professionally recommended guidelines for library practice need to be studied in the context of real work, and called for "further studies observing and comparing what those who call themselves 'information professionals' actually do in practice." A small number of researchers have recently begun to consider the contribution of more than two people to the reference transaction. Melissa Gross's work on the imposed query (Gross 1995, 1998, 1999) acknowledges that the person asking a reference question–the *agent* (Gross and Saxton, 2001)–might not necessarily be the person wanting the answer–the *imposer* (Gross and Saxton, 2001). Gross (1998) offered suggestions for providing effective reference service for imposed queries and emphasized the importance of good question negotiation.

Less attention has been given to reference transactions in which more than one staff member is involved. Several writers have made recommendations about staff collaboration in the reference transaction. Kemp and Dillon (1988) discussed the value of staff collaboration as a strategy for improving the accuracy of reference service. Nolan (1992) advised that collaboration with a colleague, referral at the end of a reference transaction, and peer coaching are among the practical steps that staff could take to improve reference performance. Several of the Reference and User Services Association (RUSA) *Guidelines for Behavioral Performance of Reference and Information Services Professionals* (American Library Association, 1996) address consultation (e.g., Guidelines 4.8 and 5.4) and referral (e.g., Guidelines 4.17, 5.6, 5.7, and 5.8). Quinn (2001) considered relations between staff members in "double coverage" situations, in which more than one librarian is working at the desk at the same time. He reviewed the sociology and psychology literature on cooperation and competition, and made recommendations about using the findings from other disciplines to enhance relations between staff members working at the reference desk together. Quinn (2001) observed that "there is an implicit assumption that the two librarians may collaborate at times and assist one another in answering questions, thereby enhancing the quality of the reference service." He suggested that a study of cooperative and competitive behaviors are important because "a strongly cooperative relationship between two librarians can have a profound effect both on the quality of librarians' working lives and on the quality of reference services that the user receives . . . It is the user who ultimately stands to lose the most when librarians are unable to relate well to one another at the desk" (Quinn, 2001). Apart from Radford's (1998) analysis of the factors users rely on when choosing between staff members at the reference desk, however, it does not appear that multi-staff transactions have been studied systematically.

This paper contributes to the literature on the evaluation of user satisfaction with the reference transaction (Durrance, 1989) by reporting on data collected from users' descriptions of public and academic library reference transactions in which more than one staff member played a part. In some cases, users described these contributions as quite helpful to answering the question. In other cases, staff interaction was represented much less positively. This paper analyzes the characteristics of effective and ineffective staff consultation and collaboration in users' accounts and suggests ways that guidelines for effective reference desk behavior might be extended to accommodate situations with more than one staff member.

DATA COLLECTION

Since 1982, students in the Information Sources and Services course in The University of Western Ontario's MLIS program have completed a practical assignment in which they describe in detail their experiences as users of reference services. Students ask a personally relevant question at a reference desk in a public or academic library. The assignment report consists of an account of what happened during the library visit. Students are instructed to "include everything you did, said, and thought as well as everything that others said and did" and are asked to reflect on how they felt throughout the encounter, and on what was helpful or unhelpful. In addition, students complete a brief questionnaire in which they specify the kind of library they visited, and rate reference staff friendliness and understanding of the question, helpfulness of the answer, satisfaction with the experience as a whole, and whether they would return to this staff member for another question.

To date, nearly 300 students have contributed their "Library Visit Reports" for ongoing faculty research. These reports, and similar assignments conducted at other library schools (Baker and Field, 2000), have provided the raw material for a number of analyses of effective and ineffective elements of the reference transaction (Ross and Dewdney, 1994, 1998; Dewdney and Ross, 1994; Ross and Nilsen, 2000). This article is based on an analysis of the 237 accounts collected between fall 1998 and spring 2001.

It is important to bear in mind that the data analyzed for this study consist of students' *accounts* of their reference encounters, not transcripts of the encounters themselves. It is possible that other students interacted with more than one staff member but neglected to describe this interaction in their reports. In addition, Dewdney and Ross (1994) observed that students completing this assignment described encountering a "lack of identifying cues by which professional librarians could be identified." Although student accounts almost universally speak of "librarians," it is likely that many of these encounters involved paraprofessional staff.

FINDINGS

Of the 237 accounts collected during this time period, 109 (46%) mentioned more than one staff member. The majority of these accounts (81, or 74% of multi-staff accounts) report the presence of more than one staff member but provide little detail. In some cases (36, or 33% of multi-staff descriptions), students simply mentioned that more than one staff member was on the desk. In others (45, or 41% of mentions of more than one staff member), they described independent serial encounters with staff members, e.g., when the user visited two different libraries or had unrelated discussions with two staff members: "After reading the article and taking notes, I asked another staff member what to do with the periodical." (Note: large public library.) As Ross and Dewdney (1998) have found, serial visits to staff members or libraries sometimes constitute a user's counter-strategy in the face of poor reference service. The present article, however, describes those accounts (37 accounts, or 33% of mentions of more than one staff member, or 15% of all accounts) that contain more substantive descriptions of multi-staff reference transactions.

Substantive descriptions of multi-staff encounters focus on three aspects of the reference transaction: the initiation of the reference encounter, collaboration between staff members, and serial encounters with more than one staff member. The remainder of this paper provides examples of these three aspects, and considers users' descriptions of the positive and negative forms of staff behavior associated with each, with a view to extending behavioral guidelines to accommodate the complexities of transactions in which more than one staff member takes part.

INITIATION OF THE REFERENCE TRANSACTION

Radford (1998) found that impressions based on the appearance and nonverbal behavior of staff members contribute to users' decisions to approach and initiate an interaction. One reason that users might choose to approach a particular staff member is that member's move to initiate an interaction. Both Dyson (1992) and Dewdney and Ross (1994) found that users consider initiation behavior (e.g., smiling, making and maintaining appropriate eye contact, greeting the user) a helpful element of a reference transaction. Both Radford (1998) and Dewdney and Ross (1994) identified staff conversations as a potential barrier to approachability: "The staff member . . . kept me waiting for several minutes while she talked to other librarians at the desk" (Dewdney and Ross, 1994). What do users describe as positive and negative elements of approachability in a "double coverage" (Quinn, 2001) situation?

As might be expected from the findings of other studies, students described staff conversations unrelated to their question as unhelpful:

> She went back to the rear office and chatted away with the other employees. Actually, they were not all too quiet because I could basically decipher what they were saying. I don't believe that the library has to be a stale environment, but I must admit it did distract me a little from my search . . . When I walked over to the desk once again all three of the employees in the back turned and looked at me. They conversed about who would be the one to tend to me, and eventually one of them approached to find out what I wanted. (Note: branch public library.)

Likewise, users described initiation behavior such as smiling, making eye contact, and finishing other conversations as positive elements:

> There were three librarians working at the desk, two of whom were busy with other patrons. The librarian who helped me was sitting, but he noticed that I was looking to be served and he came over to me immediately. (Note: large public library.)

> Here two librarians, a man and a woman, both middle aged, were sitting face-to-face, talking. As soon as they spotted me they stopped their conversation and turned to face me. Neither of them smiled, but they looked interested in my direction. Something in their eyes gave me the impression that they were willing to help me. I thought that the direct eye contact, the fact that they were squared to me as well as the fact they stopped talking as soon as I approached was much more welcoming than my first encounter. (Note: large public library.)

In addition, some users described situations in which staff members initiated interactions with users not yet acknowledged by their colleagues:

> Standing in line, waiting to ask the reference librarian for help, another one approached asking if help was needed. I found this to be very positive as in most of my experiences in libraries it is usual to have to "wait your turn" rather than have the help come to the user. (Note: main academic library.)

Additional factors, however, contribute to approachability when more than one staff member is involved in acknowledging a user. In each of the following descriptions, one staff member appropriately acknowledged the user, but the user described the encounter negatively:

> After a few seconds a man who was sitting in the adjoining office looked at me but did not come out. A few seconds later a second man came to the desk and asked how he could help. I did not wait long, but the hesitation was long enough that I interpreted that it was not the first person's turn to help, and that he was waiting for the second to take his turn. This made me feel as though I were an unwanted task. (Note: subject or departmental academic library.)

As I approached the reference desk, I observed two women behind it. One seemed occupied with sorting, opening, and piling mail according to types of media. The other woman . . . busied herself at the computer on the desk in front of where she stood. I approached the desk, my question ready and smiled. The woman with the mail looked up and smiled briefly, then returned to her work–obviously I was not her responsibility, I thought. I turned toward the woman at the keyboard and again smiled and waited for her to notice me. Her eyes continued to scan the screen, her fingers jabbing at the keys, for approximately two minutes before she looked up at me and asked, "Can I help you with something?" Her tone implied that I was taking her away from something very important, although a quick survey of the library indicated that I was the only one in there. (Note: branch public library.)

With a single staff member at the desk, appropriate acknowledgment indicates availability and willingness to provide service. When more than one staff member is present, initiation may be more complex: the non-serving staff member may acknowledge the user when the serving staff member does not. Users described this form of acknowledgment as distinctly unhelpful. Staff members who attend to one another's approachability as well as their own could ensure that users feel appropriately acknowledged in double coverage situations.

COLLABORATION

Consultation among staff members has been advocated as a means of improving reference performance for more than 50 years. Margaret Hutchins' 1944 *Introduction to Reference Work* advises the librarian what to do when all individual efforts to answer a reference question have failed:

[S]hould he then give up? No, he should call on other members of the staff for suggestions. Any one of them may have some additional information on the subject which furnishes material on which to base another hypothesis. In some cases another staff member may know just where to lay his hand upon the very thing. (Hutchins, 1944)

RUSA Guideline 5.4 (American Library Association, 1996) encourages staff members to "consult other librarians when additional subject expertise is needed." There has been little mention in the library and information science literature, however, of how such consultation, in which the staff member serving the user consults with a colleague but remains involved in the transaction, might operate in practice. Some students completing the library visit assignment commented positively on consultations:

> [S]he telephoned two other local libraries to see if they might have something to assist my research. She let me behind the counter to talk to one of the librarians she called. He was also very helpful. (Note: subject or departmental academic library.)

> Her next course of action was to look for a librarian who specialized in government documents and who may have a better idea of where to search. She returned with a book listing all consulates in Canada and gave me the contact information for the Japanese consulate in Toronto. She also suggested, on the advice of the other librarian, that I check with Canada Post to ensure that my package can be mailed legally. I found this a very useful suggestion as I otherwise may never have thought of it. (Note: main academic library.)

> When I had wandered away from the reference desk to peruse the books the librarian had given me, I noticed that both she and her colleague were still discussing my question. One of the librarians actually went to the trouble of bringing further reference materials directly to me. This sort of behaviour made me feel that my query was a valid one and that future visits to the public library would be similarly positive experiences. (Note: large public library.)

In fact, one user identified a failure to consult as an unhelpful behavior.

> Behind the circulation desk in the glassed office sat a few women working. The woman at the circulation desk did not make any move to consult her colleagues in that office. I guessed that either she felt she had done her job by referring me to the Main Library or she felt that no one there could have been of assistance. I know that the [local newspaper] publishes the odd article on girls' hockey and that one had been in relatively recently, and in depth, about

girls' hockey in [city]. If any of those women behind her had a daughter playing hockey in [city], they would have seen the article and been able to refer me to newspaper files at least. (Note: branch public library.)

Although students' accounts provided many positive examples of consultation, descriptions also contained two negative themes. First, some students described the consulting staff members as taking over the search from the user:

> The man who was serving me did not smile, and did not say anything to me. He went back into the office area. I heard him say "funeral homes" to the first man (the one who had seen me first but had not come out). I heard the first say "Arbor" and "Loewen" and spell them for the man who was serving me. He then came out to the desk and showed me the names in a book. (Note: subject or departmental academic library.)

In evaluating the experience, this student observed that although the staff member found the answer to the question, "I did, however, feel excluded from the process of my search." Another student used similar language:

> She called over the other librarian again and he told her they didn't have the *Globe and Mail* index on that database. This made me start to doubt her competency . . . The other librarian did suggest I check the *National Post* from last Sunday . . . That wasn't what I was looking for, but for some reason I went along with her when we searched the *National Post* index in the database. I'm not a very assertive person, but I think by this point I had felt that the whole search was out of my hands anyway, that she had somehow taken over. (Note: main academic library.)

In other cases, users described consultations in which they were or felt completely abandoned by staff; one student described being "dumped" after a staff member called on a colleague for consultation:

> This colleague said that . . . he was going to dinner and had to tell the person who was helping me a few things. Without a word to me from either of them they began walking the other way, leaving me alone. I decided to find a computer and try out the URL to see if he would seek me out to offer the promised help; he didn't. After tin-

kering with the database for a little while I decided to leave. I could see the person who had been helping me still at the desk and helping others . . . I found it most upsetting that he dumped me at the end to follow his colleague. If he had said "excuse me I'll be right back with you" or even had sought me out after to make sure I was finding what I needed would have been helpful; leaving me to figure it out on my own was not helpful. (Note: subject or departmental academic library.)

Positive appraisals of collaboration included descriptions of more than one staff member attending to the user's needs and ensuring that she felt involved. Students described collaboration both when the primary staff member consulted with colleagues and when another staff member intervened after overhearing the reference transaction:

The librarian took a few seconds to consider my question. She frowned and looked at the ceiling. Apparently, the other librarian had also been listening to my question because both said, at the same time, "You should try over in the other wing. They deal with sports and stuff like that." (Note: large public library.)

Another librarian who was passing by also verified this with a nod, as I must have looked a little surprised . . . (Note: large public library.)

This "eavesdropping" practice was often described positively.

There were three librarians at this particular desk. One was helping a patron and the other two were talking amongst themselves about something work related I believe. The librarian who was standing up looked at me and waited for my question . . . She went over to the reference shelf behind the desk and picked up a book. The librarian to whom she was previously speaking stood up and suggested another book. I heard her say that this book would be easier to understand. The librarian who was helping me found the appropriate pages in both of the books . . . I agree that the second librarian was right about the books she had suggested being more helpful. It was easier to understand than the other one because it took a less technical slant, but it still provided an adequate overview. (Note: large public library.)

In one case, however, a student commented that an eavesdropper might be communicating a value judgement about the reference question:

> Another staff member who came to stand beside her at the counter looked very nonplussed about the fact that I was asking for lesbian and/or gay materials for children. (Note: large public library.)

Finally, when additional staff members took part in a reference transaction, either as a result of being consulted or of intervening of their own accord, users sometimes described the transaction as a true team effort. One student commented that "I liked that during this time, there was a co-operative atmosphere among librarians and her colleagues kept asking, 'Do you need anything?' There was a definite team atmosphere at the reference desk" (Note: main academic library). Students' descriptions of team reference encounters mentioned the complementary characteristics that each staff member brought to the encounter.

> She began to move towards a second librarian who was positioned at the opposite side of the reference desk. She then asked them to help: "Do you know how we can find a directory or catalogue of companies in Canada who currently perform online publishing services?" The second librarian replied, "I know directories of this kind exist because I've looked for one before." As we spoke, the second librarian walked to a second OPAC terminal behind the reference desk and began doing an OPAC search independent of the first reference librarian and me. In less than two minutes, the second librarian called us over to the terminal on which he was working. Without looking up, he showed us the call number, title, and location of a hard copy directory . . . of Canadian online publishers.

In reflecting on this visit, the student contrasted the two staff members' interaction styles: "The first librarian's communication skills were very good. Her courteous, friendly manner showed a refreshing willingness to help. She showed a clear understanding of my question. This understanding was evident in the Internet search she demonstrated to show me how to answer the question independently as well as her rephrasing of the question to the second librarian." The second staff member

> had anticipated my need for information of this kind and was able to answer my question very efficiently . . . This librarian provided

me a complete answer to my question that was as current as possible . . . However, he was not as friendly as the first librarian was and he communicated less effectively . . . In conclusion, by working together, the two librarians were very helpful. Through her dialogue with me, the first librarian successfully determined exactly the type of information I requested. Through his OPAC search, the second librarian did a good job of finding that information. (Note: main academic library.)

The most complex account of an encounter with multiple reference staff described a student's interaction with eight staff members as she attempted to find out about making armor at a library with a reception desk and two reference desks. The excerpt below is taken from the student's report of what happened when she approached the reception desk with her question.

Librarian #1 looked stunned for a few seconds and stared at me for a full minute before replying . . . "Try over there" (pointing to the reference desk on the left) . . . I walked over to the reference desk and said to Librarian #2, "Hello, I am looking for some information on how to make armour." Librarian #2 smiled and stared at me thoughtfully for a few seconds . . . She looked over at a librarian sitting near her (Librarian #3) and said, "Armour?" (I felt that maybe I had gone to the wrong place.) Librarian #3 gazed at me and asked, "What kind of armour, chain or plate?" (I felt hopeful, perhaps this librarian could help me since she had asked me a question to help me refine my search strategy) . . . Next she said, "Wait, go ask at the other reference desk." (I felt discouraged and confused. I was surprised that my question was so difficult and I was unsure if there was any point in going to the other reference desk.) . . . I walked across the library to the second reference desk and said to Librarian #4, "Hello, I am looking for some information on how to make armour." . . . Another librarian (Librarian #5) came over to help me, having overheard my discussion with Librarian #4 . . . Librarian #4 turned to Librarian #6, who was obviously her supervisor, and asked, "Do you know if we have any books on how to make armour?" . . . Librarian #6 left and simultaneously, another librarian (Librarian #7) entered into the search. She typed into her computer and said to everyone in general, "Maybe I could call Mrs. X at [another library branch]." She phoned. "Oh, she is not in." . . . Librarian #6 came back with a big

book called *The Complete Encyclopedia of Arms and Weapons.*
He looked at me and said, "This is a history book but it has some
pictures and diagrams that could be useful." . . . Librarian #5, who
has been typing at her computer for a while, stopped and looked at
me and said, "Here is a website on armour! Hey, it says here to
learn from your local armourer." (Everybody laughed.) Librarian
#4 then said to me, "You don't have to stand there, go sit (she
pointed at a table) and look at the reference book. We'll let you
know when we find more." (I felt discouraged and uncertain. I was
not sure if I was being dismissed or if they would really continue to
help me.) . . . After fifteen minutes had passed, Librarian #7 came
to my table and handed me a piece of paper with the words, "Artist
Blacksmiths Association of North America" written on it. She did
not say anything and walked away rapidly before I had a chance
to ask her what I was supposed to do with the information . . .
Five minutes later, Librarian #5 came over to my table. She
handed me a piece of paper and said, "Here is the website for the
SCA [Society for Creative Anachronism, which had been discussed earlier]." . . . After Librarian #5's rapid departure, another
librarian (Librarian #8) came over to me. She smiled and said,
"Hello, are you the person looking for information on how to make
armour? (She handed me a note.) This is, or at least was, the person
in the SCA who handles new members. If she isn't, she will still
know who to forward you to. If you have any other questions,
please call me." (She handed me her business card. I felt positive.)
. . . A few minutes later, Librarian #4 came over to my table. She
said, "If you would come to the computer over here, I found a
website on armour making." . . . (The website was excellent, it had
patterns, instructions, and links to other sites. I felt elated. Finally,
after a frustrating search, I had the information I was looking for.)
Finally, as I was getting ready to leave, Librarian #2 came over to
me and said, "I found a book with pictures of armour in it, a cos-
tume book. I don't think it's what you wanted (she trailed off) . . ."
(I felt surprised that Librarian #2 had remembered my question
and that she had come to look for me after sending me to the other
reference desk.) I replied, "Thank you but Librarian #4 found a
great website for me. I am all set to make armour now!"

In reflecting on this experience, the student wrote "I was particularly
impressed by the manner in which all of the librarians worked together
as a team. For example, although I had asked Librarian #4 my question,

Librarians #5-#8 immediately became involved to assist her once they realized she was having difficulty." Although this was the only account of such complexity, many of the positive and negative elements included in it (e.g., remembering the question, including the user) are recognizable from general guidelines for reference performance (Dyson, 1992; American Library Association, 1996; Dewdney and Ross, 1994). In transactions involving several staff members, reference staff might consider attending to the ways that they interact with one another in addition to the patron, and might look for ways of systematically drawing on colleagues' complementary strengths.

SERIAL INTERACTIONS

Several writers have noted the effectiveness of monitored referrals, when a staff member sends a user off to another location and invites him or her back for a follow-up in case the referral is unsuccessful (Dewdney and Ross, 1994; RUSA Guidelines 5.2, 5.3, American Library Association, 1996). Student accounts analyzed for this study provided examples of monitored referrals:

> He then wrote down the title of the book and its call number on a small sheet of paper and gave me directions to the reference desk on the second floor. "If they can't help you upstairs just come back down here and we'll have a look in some of the Canadian encyclopedias." (Note: large public library.)

However, students described an additional element of a successful referral, in which the first staff member takes some action to ensure that staff in the referral location are available and able to address the user's question (see RUSA Guidelines 5.6, 5.7, American Library Association, 1996):

> The lady stepped from around the desk. She seemed to be looking at someone. Then she turned back to me and said, "You see that silver pole in the middle of the floor, there is a lady sitting at the desk there. Ask her for what you want." I thanked her and walked towards the pole. Not until I was almost at the pole did I see the person at the desk. As I got close to the desk the librarian raised her head from what she was doing and asked, "May I help you?" (Note: branch public library.)

When I was about to leave her desk she asked me to wait for a moment, so that she could phone somebody upstairs looking after "multilingual collections." She talked to somebody over the phone for a few minutes, and informed me that the library has no books in Bengali in its collection . . . When I approached the information desk upstairs I found two persons working there. I asked one person whether she got a phone call from downstairs a few minutes ago about the multilingual collections. The other person said that she was the one who had the phone conversation, and came forward to answer my questions. (Note: large public library.)

I could see that Carolyn was trying to help me in various possible ways. Carolyn and I returned to the reference desk. She again mentioned that this was a challenging question for her. She wanted to continue her search under CBCA full-text database. Unfortunately at this point she had to leave for a presentation. But before she left she asked Debbie, her colleague, to help me out. Debbie was even more enthusiastic about this search than Carolyn.

In commenting about the experience, this student said: "I would definitely say that this was a very positive library visit experience. What impressed me about this visit was the friendliness and professionalism of those two librarians, and their eagerness to satisfy their patron, the user . . . In working together, both Carolyn and Debbie displayed a spirit of good teamwork" (Note: main academic library).

These consultative referrals, in which the first staff member verifies the availability of other staff members, perform some of the same functions as monitored referrals–they enable the staff member to be relatively certain that the user will successfully continue the reference transaction with another staff member. In addition, the consultative referral may allow the user to avoid having to explain the question and the search process to new staff members, a process that some users described as unhelpful:

I was also disappointed that I had to tell my story several times to different people. While I did have to move from one area of the library to another (from reference to vertical files), this transition could have been better handled by escorting me, and explaining my information request. (Note: large public library.)

Students provided a number of negative examples of the referral, particularly in the context of staff turnover at breaks or at the end of desk shifts:

> There was a lady and a gentleman behind the desk. She was at the front counter adding up a tally sheet so I approached her. I said, "Hi, I was wondering if you could give me a hand finding information on the Landlord and Tenant Act." Her reply was rather unprofessional. She huffed and said, "Well, I'm finished," and then said to the gentleman, "Landlord and Tenant Act." This really made me feel insignificant and that helping me wasn't important to her now that her shift was over. I understand her passing my inquiry on to someone else, however, she could have said something like, "I can't but 'Bob' can. 'Bob,' this young lady is looking for information on the Landlord and Tenant Act." This would have been more professional and still make my question seem important. Her handing me off was helpful because she did not seem like she was interested in helping me, and "Bob" was ready to lend a hand. (Note: main academic library.)

> The librarian then goes and gets a reference book. Another woman approaches her and tells her that she can go on her break. She questions what it is she is working on. They both leave the counter and discuss the contents of some file sitting on a desk. I am starting to get annoyed. While they are having their conference, I overhear three other staff members (who are also behind the counter) gossiping about a colleague who had just left the scene. I find this very unprofessional and proceed to glare at them. The two librarians return to me and Librarian #1 explains my request to Librarian #2 . . . Librarian #1 goes on her break. Librarian #2 goes to look through the reference book *Chase's 1999 Calendar of Events*, but is approached by another librarian (the one who was being gossiped about). They have a personal chat (lasting approximately one minute). I find this very rude. (Note: large public library.)

There are several situations in which a staff member will need to "hand a user off" to a colleague, and both hand-offs and consultative referrals are forms of staff collaboration that deserve more attention. Student descriptions of hand-offs emphasized the helpfulness of explaining to the user what is happening and why, verifying the availability of the second staff member, and/or accompanying the patron to the second staff member (see RUSA Guideline 5.7), and communicating with the second staff member to explain the question and describe what has been done so far to answer it (see RUSA Guideline 5.6), and the unhelpfulness of using the hand-off as a chance to catch up with a colleague.

CONCLUSION

Users' accounts of reference transactions involving more than one staff member reinforce the appropriateness of many accepted guidelines for reference desk behavior created within the "one user, one staff member" model of the reference transaction. In addition, however, these accounts suggest situations that are not so well reflected in practice guidelines. If the proportion of student accounts mentioning more than one staff member (109 of 237, or 46%) is representative of the number of such transactions in practice, it would be valuable to rethink traditional assumptions about the one user/one staff member model. Gross (1995, 1998, 1999; Gross and Saxton, 2001) has begun to analyze the implications of multiple users in a single reference transaction, and this study introduces some of the characteristics associated with the presence of multiple staff members.

Further research is needed into several aspects of the multi-staff reference transaction. Radford's (1998) work on initiating the reference encounter has provided a beginning for re-evaluating the practice guidelines for approachability, interest, and listening/inquiry when more than one staff member is involved. Other studies of effective reference communication (Baker and Field, 2000; Dewdney and Ross, 1994; Dyson, 1992; Ross and Dewdney, 1994, 1998; Ross and Nilsen, 2000) draw attention to effective elements of staff collaboration in the search process, and effective referrals as part of appropriate follow-up. Students' accounts of their reference transactions with more than one staff member, however, describe a number of elements that require more attention, both from researchers and from professionals.

REFERENCES

American Library Association. Reference and Adult Services Division. Ad Hoc Committee on Behavioral Guidelines for Reference and Information Services. (1996), "Guidelines for Behavioral Performance of Reference and Information Services Professionals," *RQ* 36 (Winter), 200-203. Also available at: http://www.ala.org/rusa/stnd_behavior.html.

Baker, Lynda M., and Field, Judith J. (2000), "Reference Success: What Has Changed over the Past Ten Years?" *Public Libraries*, 39 (January/February), 23-27.

Chelton, Mary K. (1999), "Behavior of Librarians in School and Public Libraries with Adolescents: Implications for Practice and LIS Education," *Journal of Education for Library and Information Science*, 40 (Spring), 99-111.

Dewdney, Patricia, and Ross, Catherine Sheldrick. (1994), "Flying a Light Aircraft: Reference Service Evaluation from a User's Viewpoint," *RQ*, 34 (Winter), 217-30.

Durrance, Joan. (1989), "Reference Success: Does the 55% Rule Tell the Whole Story?" *Library Journal*, 114 (April 15), 31-36.

Dyson, Lillie Seward. (1992), "Improving Reference Services: A Maryland Training Program Brings Positive Results," *Public Libraries*, 31 (September-October), 284-89.

Gross, Melissa. (1995), "The Imposed Query," *RQ*, 35 (Winter), 236-43.

Gross, Melissa (1998), "The Imposed Query: Implications for Library Service Evaluation," *Reference & User Services Quarterly*, 37 (Spring), 290-99.

Gross, Melissa (1999), "Imposed Queries in the School Library Media Center: A Descriptive Study," *Library & Information Science Research*, 21, 501-21.

Gross, Melissa, and Saxton, Matthew L. (2001), "Who Wants to Know? Imposed Queries in the Public Library," *Public Libraries*, 40 (May/June), 170-176.

Hogan, Donna R. (1996), "Cooperative Reference Services and the Referred Reference Question: An Annotated Bibliography 1983-1994," *Reference Services Review*, 24 (Spring), 57-64.

Kahn, Leslie. (2000), "Pressing the F1 Key—and Finding Each Other," *The Reference Librarian*, no. 67/68, 99-110.

Kemp, Jan, and Dillon, Dennis. (1989), "Collaboration and the Accuracy Imperative: Improving Reference Service Now," *RQ* 29, (Fall), 62-70.

Nolan, Christopher W. (1992), "Closing the Reference Interview: Implications for Policy and Practice," *RQ*, 31 (Summer), 513-521.

Quinn, Brian. (2001), "Cooperation and Competition at the Reference Desk," *The Reference Librarian*, no.72, 65-82.

Radford, Marie L. (1998), "Approach or Avoidance? The Role of Nonverbal Communication in the Academic Library User's Decision to Initiate a Reference Encounter," *Library Trends*, 46 (Spring): 699-717.

Reference Services Review. (2001), Special issue on Faculty-librarian partnerships, v. 29, (2).

Ross, Catherine Sheldrick, and Dewdney, Patricia. (1994), "Best Practices: An Analysis of the Best (And Worst) in Fifty-Two Public Library Reference Transactions," *Public Libraries*, 33 (September/October), 261-66.

Ross, Catherine Sheldrick, and Dewdney, Patricia. (1998), "Negative Closure: Strategies and Counter-Strategies in the Reference Transaction," *Reference & User Services Quarterly*, 38 (Winter), 151-63.

Ross, Catherine Sheldrick and Nilsen, Kirsti. (2000), "Has the Internet Changed Anything in Reference? The Library Visit Study, Phase 2," *Reference & User Services Quarterly*, 40 (Winter), 147-155.

A Product of Social Interaction: Tag-Team Reference and Workplace Relationships

Michelle S. Millet

SUMMARY. Interacting socially with colleagues creates close workplace relationships. These relationships translate into a dynamic, synergistic environment at the reference desk, also known as tag-team reference. When two people work well together, they can bounce ideas off of one another and serve the users most efficiently. Reference librarians all have strengths and weaknesses and those who work closely together can rely on each other without worrying about the stigma of reference desk boundaries. While traditional training and advice literature do not stress the importance of workplace relationships, there are ways that librarians and libraries can successfully promote social interaction and nurture a collaborative, collegial environment. *[Article copies available for a fee from The Haworth Document Delivery Service: 1-800-HAWORTH. E-mail address: <docdelivery@haworthpress.com> Website: <http://www.HaworthPress.com> © 2003 by The Haworth Press, Inc. All rights reserved.]*

KEYWORDS. Interpersonal relations, social interaction, reference, collaboration, competition

Michelle S. Millet is Assistant Professor, Information Literacy Coordinator, Elizabeth Hugh Coates Library, Trinity University, One Trinity Place, San Antonio, TX 78212-7200 (E-mail: michelle.millet@trinity.edu). At the time this was written, she was Reference Librarian and Outreach Coordinator at the Maureen and Mike Mansfield Library of The University of Montana, Missoula, MT.

[Haworth co-indexing entry note]: "A Product of Social Interaction: Tag-Team Reference and Workplace Relationships." Millet, Michelle S. Co-published simultaneously in *The Reference Librarian* (The Haworth Information Press, an imprint of The Haworth Press, Inc.) No. 83/84, 2003, pp. 23-31; and: *Cooperative Reference: Social Interaction in the Workplace* (ed: Celia Hales Mabry) The Haworth Information Press, an imprint of The Haworth Press, Inc., 2003, pp. 23-31. Single or multiple copies of this article are available for a fee from The Haworth Document Delivery Service [1-800-HAWORTH, 9:00 a.m. - 5:00 p.m. (EST). E-mail address: docdelivery@haworthpress.com].

Digital Object Identifier: 10.1300J120v40n83_03

Working in an academic library has taught me a great deal about what I know and, more importantly, what my colleagues know. Much of what I have learned from my fellow librarians at The University of Montana comes from interacting socially with them. While at the desk, sitting within a few feet of each other, two individuals can usually overhear each other's reference interview. Often, two colleagues with a good working relationship can turn to each other for help and work together on the best solution, if necessary. Within the larger context of the library, socializing with colleagues from different departments will knock down invisible barriers for everyone and also help at the reference desk. Collaboration, often the result of social interaction, creates a good working environment that benefits our users.

At the Maureen and Mike Mansfield Library of The University of Montana-Missoula we utilize an Information Center that encompasses the traditional reference desk, circulation, reserves, media materials and interlibrary loan. During fall and spring semesters, the desk is usually staffed with two people. The space is workable, yet not enormous, translating into a cozy work environment. If a collaborative relationship between the individuals working the desk exists, this set-up is a positive one and the user benefits enormously. At times, the desk is quite busy and both individuals are fielding a variety of questions: everything from "How do I write in French on Microsoft Word?" to "I need help finding some articles to write my public policy paper." Again, in an ideal work environment, with two professional collaborators behind the desk, we can utilize each other's strengths. We all have different areas of interest and expertise and being able to recognize and make the most of that knowledge creates what I have dubbed "tag-team reference."

TAG-TEAM REFERENCE, COMPETITION AND COLLABORATION

Witnessing a tag-team reference session firsthand can be an experience for the end-user, as information is rapidly digested and exchanged at the desk, in order to come up with the best solution to satisfy the user's information needs. Tag-team reference works best when the desk is slow enough that two people can help one user and when two individuals work well together. I also call on my desk colleague if I know that she can answer a question more thoroughly. Two librarians who have built that good, working relationship are not threatened by each other and can take and make suggestions. For example, in a tag-team situation where a student comes to the desk and needs articles discussing reading comprehension in the K-6 environment, one librarian can search through the *ERIC* database, while the other person can search *Education Index*. While we are looking, we can brainstorm our results aloud. If the results are still not satisfactory or the user needs more assistance, then we continue. One person will search the Internet while the other person chooses another resource. Working in tandem creates success and synergy.

Without a sense of collaboration at the reference desk, the result is often competition. Competition is embedded throughout American culture. It is what Alfie Kohn (1992) called "The 'Number One' Obsession" in his work *No Contest*. Kohn argues that we have to create organizations where people work together, instead of working in constant competition. In many workplaces, one has to outdo another person in order to achieve success, such as a promotion. Even in academia, faculty members are judged against one another for a variety of awards and work to excel in their areas of study, sometimes to the detriment of their students and organization as a whole (Frank, Levene & Piehl, 1991). Yet, in libraries, we need to be aware of the power of collaboration, how to foster it, and understand how socializing with our colleagues can help us create a collaborative workplace culture.

If two librarians at the desk do not know each other well, or like each other, then offering your assistance becomes "butting in" and "grandstanding." At the reference desk, we often try not to cross the well-established boundaries. Being able to call on a colleague, however, is pivotal to providing good service. In his article "Cooperation and Competition at the Reference Desk," Brian Quinn (2001) discussed behaviors that people possess which cause us to be competitive by nature. At the reference desk, being competitive has an obvious effect on both our working conditions with colleagues and end-users. Quinn discussed ways to foster cooperation among desk colleagues, including both cognitive and behavioral interventions. These suggestions may result in what we desire at the reference desk: synergy and flow. Synergy between two librarians at the desk creates a true understanding of how much help the other librarian needs. Taking synergy one step further, flow leads to full engagement in one's work, creating a perfect working environment for the two librarians. This perfect state of reference work will lead to two individuals bouncing ideas and strategies off of one another and working together at maximum capacity (Quinn). Flow is also what I referred to earlier as tag-team reference.

Currently, there are at least eight Public Services Librarians at the Mansfield Library and two full-time Reference Technicians who work at the reference side of the Information Center. We are fortunate to have specialists in a variety of areas that also serve as part of the Information Center team. The key, however, to accessing the knowledge within your library and serving the users most effectively is creating a collegial working environment built on social competencies and interaction with coworkers. During our desk hours, we often field questions on a variety of subjects. Librarians need to be able to freely call upon our colleagues for their expertise; otherwise our ability to serve our users becomes compromised (Frank et al., 1991).

While tag-team reference works best at the desk with the individuals who are on duty, collaboration extends beyond the desk as well. Personally, I never hesitate to call the Serials Department to inquire about a record in the catalog or consult with someone in the building that knows the answer for my user. At the Mansfield Library, we concentrate on user-focused services, which include everyone from circulation staff to librarians to technical services staff and everyone in between. Extending our social relationships beyond our department helps create those comfortable relationships that result in effective work. From the Information Center, we process rush-cataloging requests in tandem with the Technical Services Department. Again, most of my knowledge of who knows what in other departments comes from what I learn from them in personal conversations. Social interaction, in and out of the workplace, helps create a true sense of collegiality. The dilemma though, is getting our colleagues to buy in to this practice. It's not as if we were taught to socialize with our colleagues and build relationships in graduate school, were we?

SOCIAL COMPETENCIES, TRADITIONAL TRAINING AND ADVICE LITERATURE

Traditional reference training lacks discussion regarding the psychology of working relationships and effective collaboration. In one of the more popular general reference course books, no discussion of consulting colleagues occurs. Extensive dialogue exists about the reference interview, and Bopp and Smith (2001) note that successful reference "depends heavily on the ability of the library staff to conduct a successful reference interview." Good reference interviews depend upon librarians wanting to help their users and possessing the knowledge to utilize a variety of information sources (Bopp & Smith). What about the reference sources otherwise known as your colleagues? Sometimes our ability to be successful at the desk depends on asking our friends at work for help.

In his article, "Using Emotional Intelligence in the Reference Interview," Marshall Eidson (2000) noted that social competencies are truly important for reference service. Utilizing the work of Daniel Goleman, Eidson illustrates that social competencies for libraries are vital to the successful reference interview. Goleman asserts that one-half of emotional intelligence includes social competencies comprised of empathy and social skills (Eidson). For the purposes of this discussion, the social skills are most critical. When helping users at the reference desk, we employ social skills and emotional intelligence on a consistent basis. They are equally important in creating a synergistic environment.

A plentiful amount of good advice literature exists for new librarians. Librarians advise their new colleagues about budgeting work and professional development (Berry & Reynolds, 2001; Locknar & Vine, 2001). Others have noted the importance of being friendly, welcoming and paying attention to public services (Leonicio, 2001). Other significant articles discuss the rigors of promotion and tenure, avoiding too much stress on the job, and exactly where to start with your new job. Susan Schweinsberg Long (1994) stresses that colleague support is vital to being a successful librarian and that networking with colleagues all over cannot be underestimated. Long's same principles apply to networking in your own building. Little of this literature suggests there are benefits to socializing with colleagues.

When consulting similar literature targeting new faculty members, advice exists on building support and collegiality, emphasizing the importance of socialization. One of the challenges for new faculty that Rita K. Bode (1996) notes is "creating enduring relationships with colleagues." Finding new friends and colleagues creates a better work environment. Bode continues, stating that truly "becoming a new colleague in a new environment thus requires socialization of faculty." This same principle holds true for librarians.

WORKPLACE RELATIONSHIPS

Cooperation between people exists in a variety of different relationships, including work relationships. At work, we cooperate on specific tasks, with both our supervisors and supervisees. While it is vital to co-operate at work, true work-related cooperation will not occur in the absence of a social relationship. Social relationships at work lead to essential interaction, including conveying information, discussion, negotiation, and providing advice. All of these essentials are influenced by social activity. That activity, which may or may not have to do with work at all, goes back into the relationship and influences the work itself. It is often the case that coworkers who socialize outside of work will often cooperate at work. Socializing with colleagues can also build friendships. People, by nature, like to talk, laugh, eat and smile with friends. The importance of this message is that this behavior is beneficial to the workplace and to the reference desk environment. The product of this behavior is "social cohesion," which results in cooperation and, often, friendship (Argyle, 1991).

Reference librarians often collaborate and work closely together, creating workplace friendships. Communication experts Patricia Sias and Daniel Cahill outlined the development of workplace friendships into three stages: acquaintance-to-friend, friend-to-close friend, and close friend-to-almost-best friend. The first stage, acquaintance-to-friend, came about because of "working together in close proximity" and "extra-organizational socializing" (Sias & Cahill, 1998). Socializing outside of the workplace is important because it can lead to stronger relationships, leading to better working conditions overall.

Communication researchers have also noted an important finding regarding work friendships, which could be particularly applicable to libraries. Communication between coworkers with personal relationships creates a non-threatening environment for new ideas and innovation (Albrecht & Hall, 1991). In today's library, we utilize new resources everyday and many of our facilities are undergoing a great amount of change. Albrecht and Hall also noted that personal relationships not only make innovation easier, but also often bring about new processes in the workplace because of the give-and-take between friends.

PROMOTING SOCIAL INTERACTION

In order to create collaboration and promote social interaction, reference librarians can work to implement formal programs in their libraries. They include the following:

- Mentoring programs: Newer librarians are paired up with senior librarians to build a supportive, collegial relationship. The pairs should be encouraged to interact with each other. Meeting even for small talk often leads to friendships and better work relationships.
- Cross training or non-compartmentalization: If we understand what each other's responsibilities are and work together, we will be more comfortable working together and willing to call on each other when necessary.
- Building Collegiality: True collegiality relies on creating more equality. Encourage librarians to work together on equal footing and increase cross training across disciplines and responsibilities.
- Other Programs: Encourage your library and reference department to hold gatherings as a way for librarians to interact socially. Good examples of these activities include departmental retreats, holiday parties or luncheons.

Cooperation in the workplace, and especially in libraries, results from understanding the psychology of human relationships, including social interaction with coworkers. While some people would suggest leaving their work at the office, I would argue that just the opposite is beneficial. Going out with your fellow librarians for dinner or happy hour in order to vent the week's frustrations is a great way to build relationships. In other work cultures, policy changes and other work issues are often discussed in after-work social settings. If you are unable to fit those type of after hours activities in, then make an effort to attend library-wide activities such as holiday parties or retreats (Varhol, 2000). At The University of Montana, our campus holds weekly happy hours with food and beverages for faculty and staff every Friday to build collegiality on campus. Many of the reference librarians and staff from the Mansfield Library also socialize over dinner, where they troubleshoot work issues.

CONCLUSIONS

Working in a reference department requires that we all learn and utilize social competencies and build cooperative relationships. At the same time, we should work to build a true sense of collegiality among the librarians with whom we work. We can accomplish this through formal programs or by encouraging socializing outside of work. Library-wide retreats, departmental outings and holiday parties are a few ways we can institute socializing into our schedules. The results of socializing with colleagues will always be a higher sense of collaboration and continued success when working the reference desk.

Ideally, socialization will create synergy and flow, or tag-team reference, which benefits all of our users. Tag-team reference allows us to collaborate at the desk and get our users most reliable information in the fastest way possible. Socialization and collaboration may also result in friendship with colleagues, creating the most positive working relationship of all. When we put our boundaries aside and work together, we build our work friendships. Working closely and socializing also lets librarians learn more about each other, allowing us to remember to consult that person the next time we have a question that they might know. The more we work to build collaboration, the less threatening our work environment becomes and competition at the reference desk dissipates. Interacting socially and building collegiality creates a good working environment for librarians and benefits our users.

REFERENCES

Albrecht, Terrance L. and Hall, Bradford 'J.' (1991), "Facilitating Talk About New Ideas: The Role of Personal Relationships in Organizational Innovation," *Communication Monographs* 58 (September), 273-288.

Argyle, Michael (1991), *Cooperation: The Basis of Sociability*. London: Routledge.

Berry, Susan Sykes and Reynolds, Erika W. (2001), "I Got the Job! Now What Do I Do? A Practical Guide for New Reference Librarians," *The Reference Librarian* 72, 33-42.

Bode, Rita K. (1996), "Mentoring and Collegiality," in *Faculty in New Jobs: A Guide to Settling In, Becoming Established and Building Institutional Support*, edited by Robert J. Menges and Associates. San Francisco: Jossey-Bass Publishers, 119-141.

Bopp, Richard E. and Smith, Linda C. (2001), *Reference and Information Services: An Introduction*, 3rd ed. Englewood: Libraries Unlimited, Inc.

Eidson, Marshall (2000), "Using Emotional Intelligence in the Reference Interview," *Colorado Libraries* 26 (Summer), 8-10.

Frank, Polly, Levene, Lee-Allison and Piehl, Kathy (1991), "Reference Collegiality: One Library's Experience," *The Reference Librarian* 33, 35-50.

Kohn, Alfie (1992), *No Contest: The Case Against Competition*, rev. ed. Boston: Houghton Mifflin.

Leonicio, Maggie (2001), "Going the Extra Mile: Customer Service with a Smile," *The Reference Librarian* 72, 51-63.

Locknar, Angela and Vine, Scott (2001), "Now What? Starting Your First Professional Academic Reference Position," *The Reference Librarian* 72, 43-50.

Long, Susan Schweinsberg (1994), "Enhancing Reference Services with the Support of Your Colleagues," *Medical Reference Services Quarterly* 13 (Winter), 69-76.

Quinn, Brian (2001), "Cooperation and Competition at the Reference Desk," *The Reference Librarian* 72, 65-82.

Sias, Patricia M. and Cahill, Daniel J. (1998), "From Coworkers to Friends: The Development of Peer Friendships in the Workplace," *Western Journal of Communication* 62 (Summer), 273-299.

Varhol, Peter (2000), "Mixing Work and Leisure: A Blurring Line," *Electronic Design* 48 (July), 161-162.

Reference Service in the Context of Library Culture and Collegiality: Tools for Keeping Librarians on the Same (Fast Flipping) Pages

Lisa F. Lister

SUMMARY. Reference desk service is the public face of our fast-changing profession. Because libraries often have numerous librarians sharing desk duty, consistent service can be a worthy challenge. Practical tools for promoting consistency (in the context of collegiality and teamwork) are explored. Library "culture" and organizational structure influences our professional worklives and personal job satisfaction. Sharing knowledge with one another and interdepartmental collaboration contributes to the advancement of the profession. *[Article copies available for a fee from The Haworth Document Delivery Service: 1-800-HAWORTH. E-mail address: <docdelivery@haworthpress.com> Website: <http://www.HaworthPress.com> © 2003 by The Haworth Press, Inc. All rights reserved.]*

KEYWORDS. Reference service, collegiality, cooperation, knowledge sharing, library organizational structure, library culture

Lisa F. Lister is Reference Services Librarian, Colorado College, 1021 North Cascade, Colorado Springs, CO 80903 (E-mail: llister@coloradocollege.edu).

The author would like to dedicate this article to her colleagues at Tutt Library, Colorado College, and to all the librarians in her past who so freely shared with her their insights and knowledge.

[Haworth co-indexing entry note]: "Reference Service in the Context of Library Culture and Collegiality: Tools for Keeping Librarians on the Same (Fast Flipping) Pages." Lister, Lisa F. Co-published simultaneously in *The Reference Librarian* (The Haworth Information Press, an imprint of The Haworth Press, Inc.) No. 83/84, 2003, pp. 33-39; and: *Cooperative Reference: Social Interaction in the Workplace* (ed: Celia Hales Mabry) The Haworth Information Press, an imprint of The Haworth Press, Inc., 2003, pp. 33-39. Single or multiple copies of this article are available for a fee from The Haworth Document Delivery Service [1-800-HAWORTH, 9:00 a.m. - 5:00 p.m. (EST). E-mail address: docdelivery@haworthpress.com].

Digital Object Identifier: 10.1300J120v40n83_04

In a world where databases and interfaces are quick-changing realities, how do we ensure quality, consistent reference service? How can we realize our potential and be the best that we can be? In these times when the meaning and matrix of our jobs as information specialists are seen critically from both within and without our profession, it behooves us all to reflect on the public face of the reference desk.

I am convinced that we can best move toward our professional goals buoyed by the supportive tide of collegiality. Sharing knowledge, collaborating, and employing practical tools that provide accurate, easily accessible information, all contribute to consistent reference service. This collegiality, in tandem with a library "culture" that honors intellectual excellence and freedom within a participatory setting, makes a firm foundation for the provision of quality, cutting edge reference service.

LIBRARY CULTURE

I have worked in three different academic libraries in my career: a public university, a rural community college, and a private liberal arts college. Although the students, faculty, and institutions varied tremendously from one another, the librarians and sense of library mission did not. All these libraries had highly participatory, gelatinous hierarchies that encouraged camaraderie. Fortunately, the library profession simply does not seem to vie with MBA programs for power-hungry, vertically-rising individuals, and this contributes to many of our library structures being more circular than pyramidal, more participatory than autocratic. "We work as partners, as members of a community. A well-functioning team builds on the strengths of its individual members and promotes an atmosphere conducive to consultation and sharing" (Echavarria, 2001). Although this participatory structure is not the case everywhere, I believe it is more the norm than not, and where it flourishes, it serves not only to enhance our professional work lives, but also to advance librarianship and its uniqueness as a profession. In all three libraries, my colleagues were a qualitative, integral part of my work experience.

The workplace structure itself can foster collegiality or its antithesis, competition and turf guarding. In the early 1990s, librarians at Mankato State University found themselves slipping into the unfortunate latter, due to an organizational structure that emphasized compartmentalization over cooperation (Frank, 1991). With thought and effort, librarians at Mankato transitioned to an environment where "group involvement has replaced isolated activity." It may benefit us to critically examine our structure and processes in order to identify changes that could foster greater workplace collegiality.

SHARED KNOWLEDGE

Librarians who have moved and inspired me have been the ones most willing to share the synthesis of their accumulated knowledge in meetings, workshops, and while at the reference desk.

Most of us are humble enough to realize that a diploma in hand is just the beginning of our learning as librarians. A large part of our education begins with our first professional job, and continues indefinitely. I was lucky that my first job as a reference librarian was in a position set up as an "internship," geared to a recent library program graduate. Although it was assumed that I would know the basics and be dedicated to the service philosophy of the profession, I was tenderly tutored in the nitty-gritty of day-to-day librarianship. At the reference desk, I stumbled, was embarrassed, found answers long after the patron left. Eventually, I became more graceful, learning the resources at my particular institution, but only after repeated use and ongoing study. I learned to ask for phone numbers so I could phone the patron after my eventual coup, which could be hours later. I felt comfortable picking the brains of experienced librarians, asking for help from my colleagues, just as we so often encourage others to ask us for help.

Lucky are our recent graduates, whether in a formal internship or not, who have such an environment in which to grow professionally. For those more seasoned, it is an in-house opportunity for giving back. We are a stronger profession when we communicate, network, and ask questions of one another.

COLLABORATION

We now need to know how to map to printers, write *html* and have a rudimentary knowledge of technological vocabulary so we can communicate with the techies who run the platforms upon which our world is based. Most of us, including myself, are willing and anxious to absorb these changes as best we can while holding fast to the service values that led us here initially. We know the organization of information and the nuances of the human interface, but today (and no doubt tomorrow) we must all know more. Reference librarians should seize the ongoing learning opportunity to embrace Windows and WAM tables, as well as bibliographic services and systems librarians among us. The public services and technical services perceived rift of the past has no place in this fresh complex world before us.

PRACTICAL TOOLS

Not unlike many reference desks at academic libraries, numerous librarians share reference shifts at Tutt Library, an academic library serving 1,900 students at Colorado College, a private liberal arts college in Colorado Springs, Colorado. These service providers include reference/liaison librarians, other librarians on staff (archivist, systems librarian, head of bibliographic services, director), and several part-time "on-call" or substitute librarians. In addition, a few support staff also work the reference desk.

On a practical level, how do we keep over a dozen reference desk workers on the same page when the pages are flipping so darn fast? How do we work together to provide the needed consistency for optimal service to our users? How can we best learn from and inspire one another? At Colorado College, we have found the following tools to be useful. I suspect that many libraries have similar means for promoting currency and consistency.

Monthly "Practicum" Sessions

All who work the reference desk are encouraged to attend these in-house professional development sessions. Agenda items are generated by e-mail in advance, compiled by the facilitator, and then we teach one another. A librarian with strengths in economics might do a short session on locating statistics. Our archivist might show us the latest additions to her web site. New databases are demonstrated and technology-troubleshooting procedures discussed. We are often provided a "heads-up" on class assignments from our liaison librarians. These practical, hands-on sessions give us a chance to focus on making the most of our resources, and help us to feel part of a reference team.

The "Reference Revelry"

As Reference Services Librarian, I produce an occasional e-publication that summarizes new policies, clarifies procedures, and reports newsworthy events, like the addition of new or trial databases. Although much of this information can be gleaned from various group minutes, this newsletter highlights this information with reference desk service in mind.

Index to the Reference Desk

Can't remember the video checkout policy? Don't know where students can get transparencies made on campus? The answer to these questions can quickly be found by using the "Reference Desk Master Index." That's right, the Reference Desk itself is indexed! If I had not worked as a freelance indexer for several years, this concept may not have occurred to me. But indexing and librarianship are partners in one greater cause: providing access.

With over a dozen librarians looking for scattered bits of information now and then, it made sense to provide a tool that served as a master finding-aid. We have several notebooks at our desk, including a Reference Manual, Emergency Manual, Database Manual, a Government Documents Manual, etc. Behind the desk, in Ready Reference, information on the college itself and the local area is kept. In a file drawer are handouts, mapped directions to other libraries and out-of-order signs. The storing and organization of "fugitive" information for reference use has been explored (Gangl, 2001) and a few libraries have some form of system in place. Most, in my experience, rely more on oral history or the hit-and-miss memory of the librarian on duty.

The Master Reference Desk Index is a one-stop tool that indexes the location of the contents of all these resources. In preparing such an index it becomes evident what information and policies are missing, unclear, outdated. Recently, I began indexing the content of our library staff web pages that provide detailed policies and procedures geared for internal use. We all make suggestions for additions and revisions, as the index is an evolving, ever-changing finding tool. New people find it especially valuable and useful.

Peer Collaboration During Double Staffing

During our busiest times, we staff the desk with two librarians. This provides the opportunity for librarians to consult with one another on difficult or multi-faceted queries. It is important to hold customer service skills in high regard during these times, and deny the temptation to turn this time into a personal chat session! Quinn (2001) explores the behavioral implications of double staffing, especially cooperation vs. competitiveness, and acknowledges its "potential for a wonderfully supportive synergy." Working on challenging questions as a duo can also provide a great opportunity to share professional knowledge between seasoned and neophyte librarians. Not only can this experience help foster and improve our individual reference skills, but in my experience, can provide for many enlightening and enjoyable reference shifts.

Orientation of New Reference Staff

New reference staff are given a basic orientation to desk procedures and policies by the Reference Services Librarian. After this, a desk rotation schedule is set up during double-staffed shifts so the new workers have the opportunity to work with a variety of reference librarians. This gives new people an opportunity to experience different personal styles and working methods. After about eight of these rotating shifts they generally move into their regular time slots.

The Social Ties That Bind

When staff can play and have fun together, the quality of the workplace experience is enhanced. Our job satisfaction improves as well as our ability to communicate with one another. Some library staff members have organized once-a-month potlucks in their homes on a rotating basis. This event, dubbed "First Fridays," allows staff an option to gather in a purely social setting. Although participation varies, it is an indication of a greater desire to foster additional social community beyond the workplace.

We also held our first Reference Retreat in the summer of 2002, which was a mix of fun, learning, and reflection. We took a simplified version of the Myers-Briggs Inventory to learn what "colors" we were in order to think about how to better communicate with one another. We had sessions on plagiarism and dealing with problem patrons, and then watched and discussed a lively video (Christensen, 1998) on providing customer service with passion.

CONCLUSION

Providing consistent, high-quality reference service is a challenge in any library. Our library culture and organizational structure can either foster or hinder the participatory ideals that contribute to our collegiality. Knowledge sharing and interdepartmental collaboration benefits us both professionally and personally. Practical tools that advance communication and teamwork can help provide needed constancy in our ever-transforming world.

So what is the public face of reference? Human, very human. Although we may sometimes falter, even fail, it is the human face of reference that has been and is now (more than ever) one of our greatest strengths. The human connections made in the course of the reference interview and ensuing shared information quest are what make our unique profession one of timeless value. To move reference service ever forward, let us trust in the powerful tide of collegiality and the brilliant beacon of our collective wisdom.

REFERENCES

Christensen, John (Producer/Director). (1998). *Fish!: Catch the Energy, Release the Potential!* [videorecording]. Burnsville, MN: ChartHouse International Learning Corporation.

Gangl, Susan (2001), "The Librarian's Library: Fugitive Reference Files," *The Reference Librarian* 72, 179-94.

Echavarria, Tami (2001), "Collegiality and the Environmental Climate of the Library," *Alki* 17 (Dec.), 22-24.

Frank, Polly, Levene, Lee-Allison, and Piehl, Kathy (1991), "Reference Collegiality: One Library's Experience," *The Reference Librarian* 33, 35-50.

Quinn, Brian (2001), "Cooperation and Competition at the Reference Desk," *The Reference Librarian* 72, 65-82.

The Reference Interview as Partnership: An Examination of Librarian, Library User, and Social Interaction

Celia Hales Mabry

SUMMARY. The reflections penned in this article began as a single paragraph contributed several years ago to Charles Anderson's "The Exchange," a column in *RQ* (now *Reference & User Services Quarterly*) (Anderson, 1995). I elaborated upon the concept through further reflection and augmented the ideas through a literature review. These ideas are meant to spark interest among library school students, new reference librarians, and veteran reference librarians who perhaps need new reason to show up with a positive attitude at that next reference shift. The thesis is that this moment in time within a given reference interview occurs only once, regardless of how many times a librarian has heard the question. We as librarians must always be alert to respond appropriately to the distinct contributions that the given library user brings to that question. In the process, we are equals in that the librarian knows more of the research technique to uncover the appropriate sources, but the library user knows more of what his specific slant on the topic will be. We would be

---

Celia Hales Mabry is Reference Librarian and Bibliographer for Reference and Religion, University of Minnesota's Wilson Library, 309 19th Avenue South, Minneapolis, MN 55455 (E-mail: c-hale@tc.umn.edu).

An earlier version of this article was published by this author on the Web under the title, "Existentialism at the Reference Desk."

[Haworth co-indexing entry note]: "The Reference Interview as Partnership: An Examination of Librarian, Library User, and Social Interaction." Mabry, Celia Hales. Co-published simultaneously in *The Reference Librarian* (The Haworth Information Press, an imprint of The Haworth Press, Inc.) No. 83/84, 2003, pp. 41-56; and: *Cooperative Reference: Social Interaction in the Workplace* (ed: Celia Hales Mabry) The Haworth Information Press, an imprint of The Haworth Press, Inc., 2003, pp. 41-56. Single or multiple copies of this article are available for a fee from The Haworth Document Delivery Service [1-800-HAWORTH, 9:00 a.m. - 5:00 p.m. (EST). E-mail address: docdelivery@haworthpress.com].

http://www.haworthpress.com/web/REF
Digital Object Identifier: 10.1300J120v40n83_05

wise to stay diligent, to listen well, and to take nothing for granted. The reference interview then becomes a lively, energetic, and stimulating discussion meant to lead to library research at its best. *[Article copies available for a fee from The Haworth Document Delivery Service: 1-800-HAWORTH. E-mail address: <docdelivery@haworthpress.com> Website: <http://www.HaworthPress.com> © 2003 by The Haworth Press, Inc. All rights reserved.]*

KEYWORDS. Reference service, reference interview, reference desk

INTRODUCTION

Arguably the most important part of reference service, if the librarian is past the initial phase of gaining her skill, is the reference interview–the way that librarian and user interact to bring about a successful experience for both. Several years ago Thomas P. Slavens (1994) wrote a definite monograph that is still useful and ought to be consulted by anyone interested in this topic. In addition to Slavens's monograph, there are a number of aspects to this relationship that have received attention in the literature over the years. The following more fully explores these aspects. User and librarian are essentially a partnership, and nothing good will ultimately come of something that is perceived in any way but equality between these two individuals, meeting in time in one moment.

There is a great abundance of scholarly analysis of the reference interview available: In the last 10 years, these authors include (in addition to Slavens, described above) Marilyn Domas White (1998); Sara F. Fine (1995); Carol Kuhlthau (1994); Catherine Sheldrick Ross and Patricia Dewdney (1994); Karen Williams, Janet Sue Fore, and John Budd (1993). (Other seminal articles are included in the bibliography.) For the most part, the philosophical underpinnings of the reference interview are not covered explicitly, and only a careful reading suggests the underlying philosophy. In this article, I would like to make explicit that which has gone unstated, perhaps because we fear that our understanding of human nature will in some way undermine our rationality and our objectivity. It is my belief that our personal philosophies (whether purely secular, scientific, religious-attuned, or eclectic) are the prime framework within which we operate, and until these concepts are examined, we will not be fully aware of why we do what we do at the reference desk. I will also argue that a model of partnership is the very best philosophy upon which to base a reference service, and to this end will draw upon the model of cooperative learning in public education that is popular in the United States.

COOPERATIVE LEARNING AND THE REFERENCE DESK

Cooperative learning is a method used increasingly in classrooms across the United States, from kindergarten to graduate school. Its chief proponents, Roger and David Johnson, have conducted extensive research across the country to prove that cooperative learning meets the needs of students better than the traditional lecture (1998, 1994, 1991, 1989). (For an extensive discussion of cooperative learning as one of the "greatest success stories in the history of educational research, " see Slavin et al., 2003.) In cooperative learning, students meet in groups to discuss the lesson, and in so doing can often learn as much from each other as from the teacher *per se*. Yet it is the teacher who guides the learning at every point.

The cooperative learning model applies well at the reference desk. The librarian currently knows more about the library, but the user knows more about his research need. As Hicks has pointed out, we work together in a "mediated" setting (1992). Working cooperatively, we will be much more likely to handle the reference interview in a manner consistent with good reference practice as well as genuine encounter on a personal level. We need to examine three areas primarily: (1) the expectations that each brings to the encounter and, particularly, how the initial interaction determines the outcome of the interview; (2) the fact that both librarian and user are actually equals in the process; and (3) the important point that we are engaging in a single moment in time that will not recur, a moment of which we are advised to consider not lightly. Many of these concepts relate to the emotional tone of the interview, and it is largely up to the reference librarian to take the initiative in adopting the right *modus operandi* in the exchange. The reference librarian is the information intermediary, the one who really makes the difference in what will result (White, 1992).

WHAT ARE LIBRARIAN/USER EXPECTATIONS?

The librarian and the user have brought to their encounter a set of assumptions that will determine the fate of their discussion. It is clear that there are steps that we can take at the outset to be sure that the encounter will work for the best of everybody involved–librarian, user, and even reference colleagues and other library users who observe the encounter. It is sometimes said that one makes an impression in the first 15 seconds of interaction; if true, it is no less true in the reference interview.

It is sometimes thought that dress, manner, and the first words that one speaks are the most important indicators of the impression that one makes. But there are many other aspects. S. D. Neill (1985) relates a complex model of user/librarian characteristics that influence the reference interview. Among these, for the inquirer as well as the librarian, are the following: character, personality, values, age, education, cognitive abilities, communication abilities and style, appearance, perception of and assumptions about libraries and librarians, etc. We will focus on appearance first.

If in an academic or school library, the librarian is likely to be less casually dressed than the user; this is frequently true for public libraries as well, but generally not true for special libraries. In that opening instant the user decides whether or not someone dressed so differently (i.e., professionally) can be on the same wave length as herself. The dress may suggest authority that will need to be de-emphasized by manner and words if the encounter is going to be empathetic.

The "manner" of the reference librarian–that she is open and approachable–is probably the most important aspect of those crucial 15 seconds. This involves body language, an open posture and an inquiring face and friendly smile. We will discuss in detail below the assertion that the librarian and user are actually equals in their exchange; yet equality of librarian and user is the most important aspect of the interaction to be made clear at the outset. Let the user know that you respect her question and that you are giving it your full consideration. Listen for the tone of the words that the user uses; if she is hesitant or timid, you must do what you can to put her at ease. You too must be at ease, to allow an answer to arise from the subconscious mind, where all that education and experience for reference work resides.

As the above illustrates, it is primarily up to the reference librarian to influence the course of the interview. As White (1981) says, the dimensions of the reference interview are "influenced by decisions made during the interview, usually by the librarian." The user will determine if he has found a sympathetic listener in you. Nearly every user wonders internally if he dares to express ignorance (which in class might get a lower grade). Is this librarian a friend to me in my information need?

Virtually none of this internal conversation is at the conscious level, but it affects the entire exchange.

The first words are crucial, in that the right type of open question will ensure that the librarian correctly elicits from the user her "real" question. Going fairly slowly at this point is recommended, because to forge ahead is almost to ensure that the wrong question has first been asked and answered, while the "real" question goes unrecognized.

As one moves past the opening 15 seconds, it is important to listen carefully, but not so carefully as to make the user uncomfortable. Also, it is quite possible that too much intensity will break your stride. One works more easily if one is relaxed enough to listen to all of the mind, subconscious as well as conscious. You will probably begin thinking of your strategy very quickly as the question unfolds. But this is not the time to jump to conclusions, because the research supports the fact that a careful interview is vital to a successful reference encounter.

Many years ago, Braun (1977) published an impressive short piece that illustrated the role of Transactional Analysis in the reference interview. This focuses on the librarian, the user, and the various ways in which the "Parent," "Adult," and "Child" interact to bring about a successful or unsuccessful conclusion. We will emphasize mostly staying in the "Adult" frame of reference, keeping the content on a rational plane. To this end, hear out the user; ask questions; move fairly slowly so that he has time to think of the right response. If you are too quick in these moments, or try to put closure on the question too early, you may find an answer, but the interview may have failed because it is not the answer that is needed. And the user may never tell you! That is how intimidating libraries and librarians can be to the typical user.

As you begin to frame an answer, let intuition rise to the surface. We all have it, even if it has been let to lie dormant in our all-too-rational world, and it can be a vital link to those storehouses of reference knowledge that have come from library school and some years of reference experience (Neill, 1985). It is likely that you will best respond to intuition when needing to know how much information to impart, and how fast to impart it, rather than what the specific information might be. Look into the user's eyes; the familiar "glaze-over" is, of course, certain evidence that you are losing her. Sometimes this intuitional response will indicate giving less information that you might think best; but it is also very possible at this point that you are giving all that the user can absorb. Each person will receive the maximum that she can at a given moment.

Your intuition can not only give you clues about the user's rate of absorption, but it will also give you hints when you are simply giving the wrong information–without realizing why consciously (Burton, 1990). Remember that we do in reference work have that research finding of approximately 50 percent inaccuracy (Benham, 1987). We can improve our average by being more attentive to the moment, conducting a thorough reference interview.

It is suggestive to realize that this encounter is not necessarily a coincidence. Why did the person select you rather than other colleagues at the desk? While it may often be that you are the available person, there are also many times when the user has a choice of whom to ask. There is something about your manner or your appearance that is attracting to this particular person.

One should note how often a question seems to be tailor-made for the knowledge that you yourself personally has. How many times has your best short-answer librarian picked up the phone and gotten the question that she is most equipped to handle? How many times have you felt an empathy for the reference question that you are asked–the reference question that picks up on your own interests and is startlingly apt for you? When one develops an easy flow in reference work, one will be aware that these types of "highs" occur daily. It is far better not to look on your reference encounters as purely "chance," but to tentatively hold the hypothesis that there is meaning to be derived for both of you from this encounter.

GETTING HELP

In the best reference settings, it is not a demerit to ask for help if one does not know where to find the answer. Cooperative reference service is the best way to go (Orgren, 1994). If this acknowledgement seems to be a demerit in your setting, then perhaps change is required. If we do not work cooperatively, asking for assistance as needed, the patron gets poor service. If we are too afraid to ask for help, perhaps because asking appears to be too threatening, then the climate of opinion in a given reference service is fearful. There are many causes for this attitude, but peer evaluations are one major cause. Certainly this method of evaluation is widely used in libraries, but if it sets up individuals as competitors in the reference process, it has gone too far.

When reference staff cooperate, the reference service is strong. Eventually we will have a truly expert group of individuals, ready to handle diverse questions. In trying to gain the courage to express ignorance about various questions and to get help from colleagues, remember that reference is set up to be a very humbling experience. We have our entire minds on the line every time that we say, "May I help you?" That takes a special kind of courage, and support from one's colleagues goes a long way toward making the pressure bearable.

The best reference librarians are keenly aware of how much they do not know, and usually they are quick to acknowledge their weaknesses (perhaps in part because of their confidence that in many areas they are strong). The reference librarian who covers for a lack of knowledge by never referring a question is frequently new to reference. Yet we must help such colleagues to feel welcome in our reference setting, and this includes acculturating them to the advantage of saying, "I don't know, but I will find out." This, after all, is the best automatic response when faced with a question that one cannot answer, and one of the best ways to learn. Such a response also does not ill-serve the reference user (Pauli, 1992).

If we take the time to think about our reference interview, it becomes obvious that we are in a teacher-learner relationship. It is not obvious, however, that we both learn from each other, and it is not obvious that what we "teach" (i.e., what we answer in the reference interview) is what we reinforce in our own minds. We are both learning from each other in every encounter, and the content of the learning is nonverbal as well as verbal. We as reference librarians also learn even better than the listener, because we are learning from our own words by reinforcement. This phenomenon is an aspect of cooperative learning that is just now being explored in education at all levels, and it is a powerful argument that the better students do not lose in a setting of cooperative learning (Johnson, 1989 and 1991).

Moreover, we are not teaching solely the content of our answers, the words that we use and their meaning; we are making an impact by the nonverbal aspects of the exchange. These nonverbal aspects frequently have a stronger impact than the reference answer itself; they correspond to the manner and style that we demonstrate. If we do not convey patience and kindness, but seem hurried or impatient, we will be "teaching" that the question (and, by extension, the user) is not very important in our eyes. What librarian wants to let such an attitude spill over to the students in an academic library, or the citizens in a public library? None! We are expressing opinions about another in virtually every nuance of our public stance; it behooves us to be as benign as possible. The content of the reference question/answer may only be the vehicle for

teaching greater truths about living–truths such as patience and tolerance. We rarely think about such intangibles in our mundane daily activities, but would we not be better off if we did think about such issues
a little more?

It is sometimes true that we look at our users with fear, and that we
impugn negative traits in them that they do not have (or if they do, that
should be overlooked). This fearful stance is caused by our sense of being threatened; it is informed, to a great extent, by projection of our own
inadequacies and insecurities. In an academic setting, for example, the
approach of a faculty member who has previously been demanding in
regard to her reference assistance will cause a tightening of emotions
and an immediate bracing for the worst (Baker, 1995). If, instead of seeing this person as a demanding and hostile user, we instead see someone
who is fearful of failing to get tenure, our attitudes will change. We will
smile in warmth, trying to assist him indeed to "make the grade" with
his peers.

It is also never helpful to attempt to correct another person who is being difficult. We do not usually do this in an obvious way, but we may
subtly express our disapproval of a public library user who seems to
have some hidden question that she does not want to share. We think,
"How can I help if she won't tell me what she wants to know?" We may
then turn testy, and this type of behavior is some of the worst that can be
observed at the reference desks across the land. (It also, not incidentally,
has the tendency to spread among colleagues, so that one testy librarian
breeds another, and eventually the service itself has taken a downward
turn.) We can abrasively ask leading questions, and then "turn off" ourselves if the user doesn't "open up" to our satisfaction. This type of behavior is quite counterproductive. Just let the person "be," keeping a
tolerant air always, seeking to answer as much of his question as the library user is willing to share. If the user recognizes that he has a friend
in you, it is almost certain that more will be shared, making it possible,
actually, to answer the "real" question. Even though you may appear to
be only helping the user in such a situation, you will actually be helping
yourself as well. Any teacher-learner situation works in both directions,
as we have suggested. What will you be teaching yourself? Certainly,
two aspects that troublesome interviews bring out in the librarian are
patience and forbearance–traits that good reference librarians always
have in surplus (Gothberg, 1987).

As the interview gets underway, and you are sorting through ways to
answer the question as well as seeking to be empathetic, always seek to
find peace in the moment. One never does her best when under pressure

that is frequently tinged with fear or anger. When relaxed and at peace, though, the encounter is beneficial to your user as well as yourself.

WE ARE ALL EQUALS

We need to emphasize that librarian and user are actually equals in the interview process. Although the librarian knows more about the library, the user is the expert in what she needs to know about the subject. This "expert" status even includes the bewildered student, who can be helped to understand her information needs by careful questioning. She may not come to the reference with a carefully-worded statement of need, but the student still has attended the class and knows more about the instructor's assignment than does the librarian. The degree of information that we have varies; yet information does not set us apart as adversaries, nor does it suggest special favor. And the student is always particularly reluctant to express ignorance, which in the classroom might mean a poorer grade from her "class participation." As Cummins says, "They [the students] must go to a relative stranger who knows things that they do not know. They must admit ignorance and ask for help" (Cummins, 1984).

Even though we have the M.L.S. and one or more other college degrees, and we have (likely) years of experience as a reference librarian, it is well to note that an egalitarian attitude works best at the reference desk. The user is not "less" than you because at this particular moment, you are in the position to be of help because of (presumably) greater knowledge. To invite the reverse attitude is to suggest an authoritarianism and an arrogant air that will undermine any empathetic attitude that might develop otherwise. At this moment, you temporarily have more, perhaps, to give than to take; but you are not superior to him. The two of you are in this together!

Moreover, you are certainly NOT the expert in what the user needs. If you even attempt to second-guess her, you will be in for rather rude awakenings. The user wants the information that she has requested; this is important. Even if you don't think that it is the "right" information; or if you think that she is taking a wrong tack, these judgments should not be the immediate part of your assistance. Sometimes you can offer a given reference book that has been asked for, and then turn the conversation to "But do you need something more specialized, or more advanced, than magazines?" You do the user a service when you acknowledge her question with a response, and then, if necessary, steer the dialogue to something that might assist more. Note the word "might"; and remember that it is up to the user to make this assessment.

Remember that in this exchange the user is "teaching" you as well. He is telling you more about particular needs, and you are learning how best to help. He is also influencing your day by the emotional tone that is being developed between the two of you. Mutually you have come together with this other person to make a change, move toward improvement of some kind, and all the while simply to enjoy each other's companionship. Anything less than this optimism will not have formed a good exchange.

As mentioned, it is truly that the "two of us are in this together." In the model of cooperative learning, teacher and student come together to learn; the teacher looks to the student's contribution as good in and of itself. The teacher is not trying to get the student to regurgitate the comments given by her as the superior in the relationship. It is not necessarily a matter of the librarian "fixing" the problem of the student–much as one might take a car to a mechanic or your body to a physician. You are there as a consultant, surely, but the contribution of the user is very, very important and will lead to the optimal outcome for the encounter (Lucas, 1993). All too often a user is likely to try to "hand over" the problem (the reference question) to the librarian and, in effect, ask her to "fix it" (provide the detailed answer to the need) without making substantial contribution at all. This is particularly true in the academic setting, when the student may not even have read her assignment very carefully, and comes with assignment in hand, so that the librarian can read it and give a "diagnosis." In the best world of reference, this simply would not happen. But since it does happen, and with some regularity, we must be ready to turn the question back to the user and ask for her best judgment about what is really needed. The responsibility is to be shared equally between librarian and user; no abdication on either side is allowed! As described earlier, the librarian knows more about the resources available in the library, but it is up to the user to know more about her particular research need as well as the particular slant to the topic that she wants to explore. So the user is teaching us as well, factually in regard to the reference question as well as in more subtle ways that approach a relationship to life itself. Obviously, this attitude does not foster a "winning" or "losing" approach to the interaction; both are equally winners or losers–depending on the success of the mutual encounter.

It is likely apparent that we are viewing librarian and user as "joined" in the sense that their goal is a shared one (to find the right information to answer the need); their emotional tenor affects each, many times in subconscious ways; and they will take away from the exchange a better attitude toward their living that day–or a mixed jumble of negative emotions that will hinder the living of the rest of the day. If you as an experienced reference librarian, think a moment about how many times an unsatisfactory exchange has colored the rest of the reference service desk slot? If you are so affected, think how much more will be the user, who is likely somewhat intimidated by the process anyway? (As we all know, many users approach a reference desk only a very few times in their whole lives.) This joining, therefore, takes many forms, but at its base is the fact that communication goes on through many channels. The right kind of communication will produce peace of mind; the wrong kind, a wastebasket of negative emotions that will include defense, attack, fear, and retaliation. Surely we want to avoid the latter and seek for the former at every possible juncture!

What aspect of interaction that we want to avoid at all costs is our own sense of judging the question, and, by extension, the user who asks that question. Judging, or evaluating the worth of a question, is absolutely none of our business! It is true that if a student has selected a point of view that will be hard to support from the literature, or (more frequently) has selected too broad a topic, we can suggest alternative ways of handling the same material. But the question itself and the person asking it need to be respected at all costs. This is particularly important when questions of religion and politics come up. It is quite typical to encounter an international student who wants to research a political question from the standpoint of his country's point of view; we will personally not always believe that various controversial stands that politicians and statesmen in various countries take are defensible, but this does not allow us to engage in influencing that student (Lopez, 1993-94). This opinion is an age-old reference maxim: Give the information asked for! And don't insert personal opinion.

Here, though, is another aspect highlighted that is slightly different from that age-old maxim. We may, like a good reference librarian, not seek to alter a person's attitude, but we may be more prone to judge it if we do not agree with it. It is very important to realize that that sense of judgment will be felt by the user, whether or not we actually say anything aloud. This is why judging another is so destructive. We certainly don't change people in this way, and we set up a situation which is adversarial. Because so much of this behavior may be subliminal, we may never realize (nor may our user) why we are having difficulty communicating. The user is likely simply to feel that she "doesn't like" that librarian. And we will feel rejected thereby. We need to give peace away, not judgment, and join with our users in a oneness that means that both of us have the same end–a satisfactory exchange that will give the user the means to find the information that she needs. To give peace away in the exchange means that we honor the exchange; we see the relationship as an "I–Thou" relationship (as Martin Buber might say) (Buber, 1970) that is respectful in the extreme. To do so may challenge us to greater acceptance than we normally know how to give, but it is a valid exercise in accepting our fellowmen and women.

Remember, too, that the individual who holds a different political or religious opinion than yourself, even an opinion that feels (to you) morally objectionable, is truly a seeker in her heart. The seeking may at times take a tack that seems contradictory to morality, but that is not for us to say. Respect the rights of others to seek in ways that you don't personally take in your life. Maybe you are wrong about your own values; or maybe you are simply actualizing a different set of values that are in no way better (or lesser) than those of your neighbors (and users). As a librarian, it is likely that you place great value on the things of the mind–the intellectual practice of book learning and greater education. Try saying that to the sports figure on campus, who has won great kudos for his athletic ability and his point-scoring! Society itself is more likely to reinforce his values than your own. This small example illustrates the dangers of expanding one's personal view to the whole wide world.

If we don't judge, if we seek always to help, it is likely that from time to time we will enjoy a brief moment in time that indeed is existential in nature. But we don't have to subscribe to existentialism to recognize that the Now of a given reference exchange is all the time that matters. If we don't answer the question well right now, there is no other opportunity. And we can't answer the question well if we are judging it or its asker. Step back and let the library user show you the way; take your cues from him; and your answers will fall more in line with that library user's real need.

THE PRESENT MOMENT IS A UNIQUE EXPERIENCE

Let us explore the thesis that the present moment is a unique experience–never before met and never to be met again. If the librarian keeps this fact in mind, she is less likely to be subject to burnout as she answers those repetitive questions.

The best way to approach the reference desk experience is to realize that you are "caught" in a series of moments of Now–a string of isolated moments in time that will never recur (Sartre, 1968). This particular instant in time is all that any of us have, but it is all too infrequently that we live in the present. For the best reference service, it is essential that we try to let go of the past and the future (i.e., one might say the past reference question and any reference questions yet to come) and focus on the particular need directly in front of you. This involves self-awareness, which Charles A. Bunge suggests is the most important antidote to the "cycle of unhappiness and frustration in reference librarianship" (1984).

How does living in the present mitigate against burnout? It is very, very helpful to recall that even though you might have answered this question (e.g., How do I find periodicals on the OPAC?) a thousand times, for the user it is the first time that he has ever asked the question. Your job is to fall in line with the emotional tone that he has, to answer as fully as possible (but not so fully as to "lose" the user), and in terms that the user seems to be comprehending. This requires much feedback from that user, and you should be attune to nuances of body language and eye contact that tell you if you are getting through at all. (We are familiar with the "glaze-over" that tells us that we have lost him! This is just the most extreme example.) If we are able to see the experience as unique for the patron and to focus on those aspects of the interchange that make it unique to you, then the interview says "fresh," challenging, and not the kind of boring interchange that cries for retirement to arrive soon! Remaining interested in one's work is a primary way to avoid burnout. It is only the stale and the stressful that moves us toward that undesired end (Miller, 1992).

Seeing the Now of reference service means that you will close off all past and close off all future during the moments of exchange with your user. Practically-speaking, you focus on her needs only, and you forget the details of what has just preceded, and you don't look ahead to what will follow. This makes for a real experience in the present, an experience tailored to what your user needs most–not by theory what you think that she might need. And, if the person appears befuddled, and unable to articulate what she needs, you quietly forgive the confusion and don't hold it against her as you try to help. You are patient in the moment, because you are not trying to get through it quickly to answer the next person in line. Remember–just this one instant–to be lived through and enjoyed! The future is only a string of these moments, and if each one in turn is handled well, the future will take care of itself. This will make all the difference in keeping reference fresh and a new experience each time that you take a turn at the desk.

In order to live in the Now, a librarian must give undivided attention to the person before him. All too often we resist this, and sometimes interrupt the user because we are pressed for time (or just impatient) and think that we have caught the gist of what he has to say. (After all, we have answered this question before!) Big mistake! The best that we can sometimes do for another is to listen quietly, and not with the intention of just waiting out the words so that we can add some of our own. Really listening takes practice, but the rewards for a reference librarian are many. All the knowledge of reference materials in the world won't solve a given user's problem if we give him books that don't meet the precise need; hence, the importance of listening carefully to determine what that precise need really is.

I also counsel listening to one's intuition in the reference encounter. If you suspect that going on and on about a given source, even though it is the "best" one, is not going to meet the need of this person, then stop! You are probably picking up on messages of body language or facial expression that tell you that you are giving her more than she can absorb, or what she doesn't really want at all! I have learned that the user usually wants to be shown, at least, the source that has been asked for. If the user comes in asking for *The Readers' Guide to Periodical Literature*, I automatically show it to her, but all the while I am plying her with more questions that might ensure that she actually gets the best tool to answer her research need. This is an obvious response, to be made on a regular basis. Intuition about the interview can take other, less obvious forms, though. Learning to listen with the inner ear is eminently rewarding, and one will find that one gives the best service when this is the habitual *modus operandi*.

SUMMING UP

With these concepts in mind, it will be clear that the interaction between librarian and patron is essentially a partnership, and nothing good will come of something that is perceived in any way but equality between these two individuals, meeting in time in one moment. We do our users a tremendous favor by "honoring" them as individuals, not seeing them as "just" so many reference questions. When we truly see another, we are open to all aspects of their interaction to us, and thus we are ready to offer the best service because we are more attuned to the whole of the encounter. We are leaving aside our personal prejudices, viewing the person with an open mind, and bringing to bear upon this moment all of our experience and education to date. It should be obvious by now that an understanding of human nature can make or break the reference encounter. Our sensitivity to these issues of partnership as equals and meeting in the present moment are a prime way to avoid the negatives that may pile upon us as we gain years of experience in the field. Living in the Now is the most powerful way to keep one's living fresh and un-tarnished by the wounds that come upon us just by living in this difficult world. Carry a bit of optimism with you as you go about your reference desk duties, and see if it doesn't rub off on your users, your colleagues, and yourself as well. Above all, keep humanistic your experience of ref-erence by concentrating on the Now as pivotal to right living in this age of conflict-ridden, technologically-oriented information.

BIBLIOGRAPHY

Anderson, Charles (1995), "The Exchange," *RQ* 34(3) (Spring): 277.

Baker, Robert K. (1995), "Working with Our Teaching Faculty," *College & Research Libraries*, 56, 379-37.

Benham, Frances (1987), *Success in Answering Reference Questions: Two Studies.* Metuchen, NJ: Scarecrow Press.

Braun, Carl (1977), "The Reference Interview," *Ohio Library Association Bulletin*, 47, 11-14.

Buber, Martin (1970), *I and Thou.* New York: Scribner.

Bunge, Charles A. (1984), "Potential and Reality at the Reference Desk: Reflections on a 'Return to the Field,' " *The Journal of Academic Librarianship*, 10, (3), 128-133.

Burton, Paul F. (1990), "Accuracy of Information Provision: The Need for Client-Cen-tered Service," *Journal of Librarianship*, 22, 201-215.

Cummins, Thompson R. (1984), "Question Clarification in the Reference Encounter," *Canadian Library Journal*, 41, 63-67.

Fine, Sara F. (1995), "Reference and Resources; The Human Side," *The Journal of Ac-ademic Librarianship*, 21, 17-20.

Gothberg, Helen (1987), "Managing Difficult People: Patrons (and Others)," *The Ref-erence Librarian*, no. 19, 269-283.

Hicks, Jack Alan (1992), "Mediation in Reference Service to Extend Patron Success," *The Reference Librarian*, no. 37, 49-64.

Johnson, David W. and Roger T. Johnson (1989). *Cooperation and Competition: The-ory and Research.* Edina, Minnesota: Interaction Book Company.

_____ and Edythe Johnson Holubec (1998), *Advanced Cooperative Learning.* 3rd ed. Edina, Minnesota: Interactive Book Company.

_____ and Karl A. Smith (1991), *Cooperative Learning: Increasing College Faculty Instructional Productivity.* Washington D.C.: School of Education and Human De-velopment, The George Washington University.

Johnson, Roger T. (1994), "David Johnson: A Leading Teacher of Cooperative Learning," *Teaching Education* 6 (2) (Summer-Fall): 123-125.

Kuhlthau, Carol Collier (1994), "Students and the Information Search Process; Zones of Intervention for Librarians," *Advances in Librarianship*, 18: 57-72.

Lopez, Annette (1993-94), "Did I See You Do What I Think You Did? The Pitfalls of Nonverbal Communication Across Cultures," *New Jersey Libraries*, 27, 18-22.

Lucas, Peter (1993), "Customer Consultation and Its Implications for Service Delivery," *Public Library Journal*, 8, 53-54.

Miller, William (1992), "Breaking the Pattern of Reference Work Burnout," *The Journal of Academic Librarianship*, 18, 280-281.

Neill, S.D. (1985), "The Reference Process and the Philosophy of Karl Popper," *RQ*, 24(3) 309-319.

_____. (1984), "The Reference Process and Certain Types of Memory," *RQ*, 23, 417-423.

Orgren, Carl F. (1994), "Cooperative Reference Service," *The Reference Librarian*, no. 43, 63-70.

Pauli, Dave (1992), "Ignorance Is Hard to Admit," *The Unabashed Librarian*, no. 85, 22.

Ross, Catherine Sheldrick and Patricia Dewdney (1994), "Best Practices; An Analysis of the Best (and Worst) in Fifty-Two Public Library Reference Transactions," *Public Libraries*, 33, 261-266.

Sartre, Jean Paul (1968), *Essays in Existentialism*. New York: Citadel Press, 1968.

Slavens, Thomas P. (1994) *Reference Interviews, Questions, and Materials*. Metuchen, New Jersey: Scarecrow Press.

Slavin, Robert E., Eric A. Hurley, and Anne Chamberlain (2003), "Cooperative Learning and Achievement: Theory and Research," in William Reynolds et al., eds., *Handbook of Psychology; Educational Psychology* (7): 177-198.

White, Herbert S. (1992), "The Reference Librarian as Information Intermediary: The Correct Approach Is the One that Today's Client Needs Today," *The Reference Librarian*, 37, 23-35.

White, Marilyn Domas (1981), "The Dimensions of the Reference Interview," *RQ*, 20, 373-381.

_____. (1998), "Questions in Reference Interviews," *Journal of Documentation*, 54(4) (September): 443-465.

Williams, Karen A., Janet Sue Fore, and John Budd (1993), "Cognitive Processes of Reference Librarians," *Research in Reference Effectiveness*: Proceedings of a Preconference Sponsored by the Research and Statistics Committee, Management and Operation of a Public Services Section, Reference and Adult Services Division, American Library Association, San Francisco, California, June 26, 1992. Chicago: Reference and Adult Services Division, American Library Association.

WORKING WITHIN THE LIBRARY: INTANGIBLES

Interpersonal Skills in the Reference Workplace

Lorraine J. Pellack

SUMMARY. Reference librarians are expected to interact effectively with a variety of clientele and are taught skills such as approachability, showing interest, and verbal and non-verbal cues. Librarians who have a knack for interpersonal skills do very well both at the reference desk and interacting with their co-workers. An area that is rarely addressed in the literature (or in library school) is that of *educating* librarians about *how* to establish professional, collegial relationships with one another. It is assumed that if a reference librarian can interact well with patrons, in a professional manner, he or she will be able to successfully "fit into" almost any reference department. This article discusses the importance of interpersonal skills within the Reference Department and ideas for improving these skills to enhance co-worker relations. *[Article copies available for a fee from The Haworth Document Delivery Service: 1-800-HAWORTH. E-mail address: <docdelivery@haworthpress.com> Website: <http://www.HaworthPress.com> © 2003 by The Haworth Press, Inc. All rights reserved.]*

Lorraine J. Pellack is Head, Science & Technology Department, 152 Parks Library, Iowa State University, Ames, IA 50011-2140 (E-mail: pellack@iastate.edu).

[Haworth co-indexing entry note]: "Interpersonal Skills in the Reference Workplace." Pellack, Lorraine J. Co-published simultaneously in *The Reference Librarian* (The Haworth Information Press, an imprint of The Haworth Press, Inc.) No. 83/84, 2003, pp. 57-70; and: *Cooperative Reference: Social Interaction in the Workplace* (ed: Celia Hales Mabry) The Haworth Information Press, an imprint of The Haworth Press, Inc., 2003, pp. 57-70. Single or multiple copies of this article are available for a fee from The Haworth Document Delivery Service [1-800-HAWORTH, 9:00 a.m. - 5:00 p.m. (EST). E-mail address: docdelivery@haworthpress.com].

Digital Object Identifier: 10.1300J120v40n83_06

KEYWORDS. Life skills, social skills, interpersonal interactions, workplace interactions, workplace behavior, staff relations, core competencies, value-added, behavioral performance, peer relations, professionalism, personal competencies

INTRODUCTION

A very eye-catching article in *American Libraries* entitled "Can't We All Get Along?" asserted that "a growing body of evidence suggests that the root cause for the epidemic of bad bosses is the growing number of problematic employees" (Manley, 1998). It seems ironic in a public service profession which stresses customer service skills and interpersonal interactions with the general public, that there would ever be a need to address interpersonal skills with co-workers. Where's the evidence that skills are poor or lacking? The fact that there are a number of library consultants specializing in organizational development such as Maureen Sullivan and George Soete implies a need for assistance in dealing with library workplaces gone awry, aka restructuring. Some of the restructuring is due to technological innovations causing workflow changes; other restructuring is an attempt to alter reporting lines due to personnel issues. Library managers are taking courses on team building, conflict resolution and facilitation skills. There are a few announcements of library staff members resigning due to workplace tensions, but even more who change jobs after only a year or two without any publicly stated reason. Interpersonal differences are often the cause, but confidentiality issues prevent these from being reported to anyone other than the supervisor and individuals involved. In 1985, *Library Literature* introduced a new subject heading for staff relations; to date, there are 110 articles with this subject heading. There are too many variations in words such as conflict, tension, getting along, collegiality, etc., to attempt to whittle the list further . . . but clearly this is the focus of the majority of these articles.

MANAGEMENT ROLE versus INDIVIDUAL ROLE

The introduction of Myers-Briggs into libraries, in the late 1980s, sensitized librarians to individual personality types and the concept that awareness of co-worker differences could help us understand and learn to work with different types of personalities. Since then, library managers have struggled to implement one management fad after another, in an attempt to improve the workplace. Rarely have workplace dynamics been addressed as the responsibility of individual employees. Managers can coach and recommend changes, but only the individual person can affect change in their behavior. It is somewhat analogous to those who promise to quit smoking or drinking–it can happen but only if they truly acknowledge the need for it and *want* to change.

> In addition to having an ethical obligation to treat colleagues with courtesy and respect, reference librarians must be able to interact effectively with one another in order to provide an optimal level of service to their clients. A well-functioning reference unit builds on the individual strengths of each reference librarian and promotes an environment conducive to consultation and sharing . . . Collegiality generated in this work environment further boosts productivity and enhances working conditions. (Jones, 1997)

As with many similar authors on this topic, Dixie Jones mainly focuses on the role of the supervisor or manager in creating a "conducive" workplace environment. Managers typically have the opportunity to evaluate and encourage employees in specific areas of need but they rarely include things related to interpersonal skill development, unless there is a large problem area. What about those employees who don't have major problems in specific areas, but might not realize they need to work on their active listening skills, or that with a little work on their persuasive skills (and some better preparation) they could dramatically improve their chances of success with a particular proposal to other librarians in Reference Department meetings? The workplace climate is not only the responsibility of the reference supervisor or manager; it is also the responsibility of each individual librarian in the unit.

REFERENCE BEHAVIOR COMPETENCIES

Much has been written about behavior of reference librarians at the Reference Desk, the reference interview, and customer service roles related to patrons. For example, *Guidelines for Behavioral Performance of Reference and Information Service Professionals* (1996) as recommended by the Reference and User Services Association (RUSA) of the American Library Association includes typical things such as approachability, shows interest, uses both verbal and nonverbal cues, etc. These are classic areas that all aspiring library school students learn, think about, and practice early in their careers. In recent years, the emphasis has been on the creation of competencies or best practices in patron interactions.

Johannah Sherrer (1996) noted, " . . . the personal attributes of librarians have a direct bearing on how effectively individual libraries move forward in providing improved, enhanced and user respected services. In any job or profession, success depends as much on attitude and approach to work as it does on training, knowledge, or appropriate degrees." Sherrer does a very good job of discussing the importance of interpersonal skills, how they impact approachability, and their relevance to a successful reference desk interaction. The appendix to his article contains an excellent "Selected Bibliography on Reference Competencies."

Mary Nofsinger (1999) wrote about core competencies, specifically related to reference librarians. Among the usual competencies related to reference skills and subject knowledge, Nofsinger also included "communication and interpersonal abilities." While most of her examples pertain to interpersonal interactions with patrons, Nofsinger concludes by saying, "each reference librarian must assume responsibility for acquiring new knowledge and developing new skills."

Unfortunately, none of these reference competencies touch on workplace skills or co-worker relations. What goes on *behind* the desk can impact approachability just as much as having a friendly demeanor when patrons first walk up to the desk. Terse comments, disagreements, and even lack of interaction between staff at the reference desk create negative tension that is noticeable by patrons and make the desk itself unapproachable. Developing/utilizing skills to assist in improving and maintaining interpersonal relations with co-workers as well as the general public is very important to creating a successful reference environment. I suggest we go one step further and expand these competencies to include behaviors related to staff interactions, both at the desk and in departmental office areas. In many cases, this may be similar to what some have labeled as personal competencies.

PERSONAL COMPETENCIES

The Special Library Association published competencies for special librarians in 1996. They divided the competencies into two sections: professional competencies and personal competencies. Personal competencies are defined as "a set of skills, attitudes and values that enable librarians to work efficiently; be good communicators; focus on continuing learning throughout their careers; demonstrate the value-added nature of their contributions; and survive in the new world of work." These skills are further defined as "creates an environment of mutual respect and trust," "knows own strengths and the complementary strengths of others," and "constantly looks for ways to enhance personal performance and that of others through formal and informal learning opportunities."

In 1999, the University of Nebraska-Lincoln libraries staff developed twelve core competencies, including interpersonal/group skills and communication skills. Giesecke and McNeil (1999) described UNL efforts in defining and creating these competencies. They defined core competencies as "the skills, knowledge, and personal attributes that contribute to an individual's success in a particular position." Interpersonal/group skills competencies are defined as "Builds strong work relationships with a sensitivity to how individuals, organizational units, and cultures function and react. Establishes partnerships at all levels and across department and functional lines to achieve optimum results." As part of this article, Giesecke and McNeil provided an appendix with interview questions aimed at identifying job candidate aptitudes in each of these areas.

These two sets of competencies are very definitely a step in the right direction. They serve as a guide for training and development of existing staff as well as areas to look at when hiring new staff. Reference librarians who have a knack for interpersonal skills do very well both at the reference desk and interacting with their co-workers. But what about those who do not have instinctively good interpersonal skills? Where do they acquire these aptitudes prior to going into the job market?

LIBRARY SCHOOL CURRICULA

An area that is rarely addressed in the literature is that of *educating* librarians about *how* to establish professional, collegial relationships with one another. Robert Stueart (1989) states his belief that teaching this concept must "permeate the whole curriculum." He stresses that students should be required to work together in groups and asserts that schools should ensure graduates understand the importance of peer relations. Levy and Usherwood (1989) first began talking about the need for library schools to develop interpersonal skills training starting in 1989. Levy was a Library Information Studies student at the time and Usherwood was a faculty member at Sheffield University. Levy later became a temporary lecturer at Sheffield and, in 1992, published a lengthy article discussing the development of interpersonal skills training integration into the LIS curriculum at Sheffield University in the early 1990s. Unfortunately, this innovation does not appear to have made the leap across the Atlantic to affect many changes in library school curricula in the United States.

ISIM University (an online-only International School of Information Management based out of Denver, Colorado) offers the *eCreation Self Assessment Survey* (http://www.isimu.edu/foryou/begin/eprocess.htm) to help individuals decide whether or not they are "suited" to a profession in Information Technology or Information Management. The survey asks about different types of work preferences and scores one's aptitude in various areas. At the end it provides a list of tasks that would be required of a person in that career and recommends comparing your work preferences to the task list to see how well (or not) you might fit. It is not a requirement for entry/exit, but merely a tool for assisting individuals in making career decisions.

I recently polled subscribers to JESSE–a library and information science education listserv–asking what types of self-assessment or interpersonal skills training are students introduced to (or required to complete) in library schools. Only three professors responded saying that they have a unit/exercise/project involving self-assessment within various classes. Others replied that their reference courses only test individual knowledge of resources; they do not test reference interview skills or interpersonal skill competencies. There is an inherent expectation that graduates from library school automatically know how to interact in the workplace and act in a professional manner. Further, it is assumed that if a reference librarian can interact well with patrons, in a professional manner, he or she will be able to successfully "fit into" almost any reference department.

PROFESSIONALISM

What is "professionalism"? Ask ten different people and you will likely get just as many different responses. Most of the articles in *Library Literature* seem strictly to equate professionalism in academic librarianship with faculty status; and in public libraries, professionalism seems to equate to staunch ethics and protection of privacy. Textbooks for library science and reference courses skirt the issue entirely or merely suggest that reference librarians should act in a professional manner; however, a definition of professionalism or professional behavior is not included. Sarah Archer (2001) tries to provide more explicit details in the scope of professionalism for reference librarians by asserting, "Professionalism can include developing basic employee skills, supporting library standards, participating in university and library functions, presenting papers, and publishing." She goes on to specify that "additional attributes include good self-esteem, a positive attitude, and a challenging plan for career development. . . . being a professional also means planning a career with continuous improvement as the goal." While Archer does not touch on what she means by "basic employee skills" and/or how they are developed, she does present a more precise picture of what it means to be a professional reference librarian. I submit that professionalism should also include standards for behavior among co-workers.

WORKPLACE MANNERS

Information on cubicle etiquette is very easy to find. One of the best write-ups I have seen is from the Monster.com Career Center (Bryant, n.d.). General workplace etiquette is much more difficult to locate and tends to vary in each workplace. Experts agree that most employees learn workplace manners "on the job" during their first few years of employment. Employees learn what is likely to please or annoy their co-workers/bosses through trial and error, and by having good or bad examples pointed out to them. This method is flawed, however, in that what may be fine in one workplace may be completely offensive in a different setting (Argyle, 1981).

Why bother with civility? Several recent articles have brought national attention to workplace etiquette, manners, courtesy, etc., and show it as a growing concern. *USA Today* reported on the results of a poll conducted in 2002 (done by Lilia M. Cortina, University of Michigan) which found that 71% of workers surveyed have been insulted, demeaned, ignored, or otherwise treated discourteously by their co-workers and superiors (Workplace Rudeness, 2002). In a study conducted by Christine Pearson, a management professor at the University of North Carolina, she asked 775 respondents to describe how they reacted to a recent unpleasant interaction with a co-worker.

Twenty-eight percent lost work time avoiding a co-worker; 22% decreased their effort at work; 10% decreased the amount of time they spent at work; and 12% changed jobs to avoid the instigator (Pearson, Andersson, and Porath, 2000). All of these are classic avoidance methods; none of these even attempts to solve the problem. Pearson recommends several prevention techniques for managers as well as tips for dealing with specific situations as they occur. Another well-written list of practical ideas for building a kinder workplace comes from Tom Terez (2002), founder of BetterWorkplaceNow.com.

> Workplace incivility isn't violence or harassment or even open conflict–although it can build up to any of those things. For most of us, it's the thousand small slings and arrows that, day after day, eat away at what Peter Drucker once called the "lubricating oil of our organizations." (Lee, 1999)

Bob Rosner (1998) agrees saying that truly off-the-wall behavior is not what is most likely to drive people to distraction. It's the small stuff–"the pebble-in-the-shoe stuff"–that relentlessly grinds down collegial working relationships. Rosner's formula for dealing with uncivil co-workers is "you can try to change them, try to change yourself, try to get help or get the hell out." The vast majority of employees try to change others or go elsewhere. In a poll conducted by *U.S. News & World Report* (Marks, 1996), 89% of respondents report workplace incivility as a serious problem . . . when asked about their own behavior, however, they were only too eager to point a finger at the other guy. Too often, it's the other person's fault.

SELF-TESTING

Try taking a close look at your own interpersonal skills and reactions. People never like to admit they might be part of a problem–let alone discover they might be lacking skills in a given area–but no one is perfect. Testing your own skills can be a very private, personal exercise in identifying your strengths and weaknesses. Once you have identified the weakest areas, set up some interventions for working on improving them.

The first step in self-testing is to be prepared for distasteful results. Often the areas in need of work are not only nonvisible, but also shocking to discover. The most common types of self-assessment tests are the following:

- Personality tests (e.g., Myers-Briggs, DiSC, Keirsey Temperament)
- Emotional Intelligence (or Emotional IQ–e.g., BarOn Emotional Quotient Inventory)
- Communication skills
- Self Esteem
- Goal-Setting
- Coping Skills
- Team Player/Building Skills (e.g., Parker Team Player Survey).

There are a plethora of interactive Internet quizzes for all sorts of skills; see the list at the end of this article for a few of the author's personal favorites. Also, try looking in a favorite web search engine using "self-assessment" and one of the above types of tests (e.g., self-assessment and coping skills). As many of the pages are likely to state, these are not all scientifically sound "complete" tests. Each has strengths and weaknesses and some are more peculiar than others; however, the results (if taken collectively) can show trends in certain areas.

Locate specific types of tests using *Tests-in-Print* or find comparative information on various tests in books such as *Psychological Testing at Work* (Hoffman, 2002). These tests are rarely free, but many are fairly inexpensive. Search the Internet for the names of these tests to see if abbreviated versions are freely available. Many companies offer "teasers" and will provide an abbreviated version to get you interested in paying for a full test with analysis of results. The best tests will also provide tips for improvement in the areas that score the lowest.

ONGOING "GENERAL" SOCIAL SKILL DEVELOPMENT

Similar to keeping abreast of current developments in the profession, librarians should also continually keep watch on possible new areas for interpersonal skill development. There are many ways to do this in conjunction with professional development such as scanning the literature and attending conferences and workshops.

Scanning current issues of various library journals can supply some interesting possibilities for personal improvement. For example, an article on "reference etiquette" in *American Libraries* (Eckwright, Hoskisson, and Pollastro, 1998) not only supplies examples of good behaviors for patron interactions, it also covers sharing questions and correcting colleagues. "Collegial relationships in a busy reference department are extremely important . . . considerate conduct between colleagues can be as important as the rules of conduct between librarian and patron." While some of the recommended behaviors may be somewhat controversial, it's a step in the right direction in that it provides suggestions for behavior in awkward situations. A keyword search of *Library Literature* on "reference librarians and evaluation" would pull up this article, but someone looking for tips on improving interpersonal skills would never locate the article without browsing the journal. *The Reference Librarian* also regularly supplies thematic issues related to competencies and reference interactions, e.g., Section 1 of no. 54 (1996) entitled "The Current State of Reference Librarianship and Competencies Required of Reference Librarians" and *Doing the Work of Reference: Practical Tips for Excelling as a Reference Librarian* (no. 72-73, 2001).

Conference presentations are, unfortunately, often overlooked by major indexing services. A very relevant presentation, "Thinking Style Preference Among Academic Librarians: Practical Tips for Effective Work Relationships" was given at the 1999 ACRL National Conference and published in the ACRL Conference Proceedings (Golian, 1999), but has not been indexed in *Library Literature*. *Library Literature* does index two reports from recent library conferences where emotional intelligence is finally being presented as an important issue for the library workplace (Flowers, 2000). The same workshop was also presented at ALA Midwinter 2000 (Rosenstein, 2000). The ALA presentation was standing-room-only and clearly shows that librarians were looking for tips on how to better manage their local work environments. These two presentations were aimed at managers to assist in improving the workplace, but since these are merely reports of presentations, they do not give the reader any detailed information from which to learn. The only way to get some of this information is by attending the original presentations. Many state and regional library conferences also provide similar types of presentations and are not indexed by *Library Literature*. It can be very expensive to attend conferences and many librarians do not get reimbursed for any of the expenses by their institutions. Those who do attend conferences should watch for these sorts of presentations and provide copies of the information to their co-workers.

LEARNING FROM MANAGEMENT FADS

Over the years, a number of fads in the business world have made their way into the library literature, particularly in library management. An excellent example of this is the emergence of the Myers-Briggs Type Indicator in library literature, starting in 1989 and continuing today (Agada, 1998). More recently, articles on the applications of emotional intelligence in libraries have begun appearing in the literature. Eidson (2000) discusses the elements of emotional intelligence and how they relate to the reference interview, but stops short of discussing their relevance to the workplace in general. Goleman (1998) defines using emotional intelligence in social skills as "handling emotions in relationships well and accurately reading social situations and networks; interacting smoothly; using these skills to persuade and lead, negotiate and settle disputes, for cooperation and teamwork." Goleman outlines a list of "social competencies"; Chapters 7, 8, and 9 deal with this topic in depth. As with any fad, they may not be applicable to reference librarians but they can generate some excellent ideas.

OTHER TIPS

Become a people-watcher. Pay attention to co-worker reactions/ questions–both in group meetings and one-on-one settings. Analyze extremely positive and negative situations looking for clues of things to emulate (positive) or avoid (negative) when interacting with specific co-workers. As reference librarians, we have learned to phrase things in ways to avoid patron angst. For example, "Is it possible you mis-typed the journal name in the search box?" instead of something like "Well of course we own that journal; you must not be searching the catalog correctly." But how often do we carefully rephrase things to avoid co-workers' "hot buttons"?

Ask co-workers to rate your skills in particular areas–pick someone you like/trust as well as one you might not get along well with. Ask for their honesty and be prepared for harsh realities in their responses. It is often difficult to accept the results graciously–but admitting the existence of faults to co-workers goes a long way toward helping and improving relations in and of itself.

Check with your institutions' Human Resources department for workshops/classes–many tailor them to specific needs/requests (e.g., working with dominant personalities, communicating without offending, etc.) or provide individual assistance in developing skills when there isn't enough call for the topic to justify a full class.

CONCLUSION

To reiterate a comment made by Dixie Jones (1997), "Collegiality generated in this work environment further boosts productivity and enhances working conditions." Traditional reference interview skills focus on approachability, friendliness, smiling, etc., to encourage patrons to ask questions and feel welcome doing so. It is frequently inferred that being in a bad mood also affects patron interactions, since it is very difficult to put on a smile and appear friendly while seething internally, but rarely does anyone state this anywhere in the literature. Similarly, interpersonal relationships among reference staff will have a tremendous impact on the service given to patrons. Interactions between staff members at the reference desk are very visible to patrons. Congeniality between staff members breeds approachability. Terse comments, disagreements, and even lack of interaction between staff at the reference desk create negative tension that is noticeable by patrons and make the desk itself unapproachable. That limits our effectiveness, gives our patrons a bad experience, and reduces the likelihood they will come back for assistance in the future. Contrary to popular opinion, old dogs *can* be taught new tricks. Interpersonal skills *can* be developed at any point in life–not just in adolescence. I submit that it is the professional responsibility of each individual librarian to continually develop and improve *personal* as well as professional competencies. Time spent developing interpersonal relationships between co-workers is a necessity for good customer service and a healthy, inviting work environment.

SOME USEFUL WEBSITES

BetterWorkplaceNow.com–http://www.BetterWorkplaceNow.com/–check out the links under "Insight and Inspiration" as well as "Laugh and Learn."

Career Planning from About.com–http://careerplanning.about.com/cs/selfassessment/index.htm.

CareerResource.com–http://www.careerresource.com/Careerplan.html–scroll down the page to a section entitled "Understanding Yourself/Self Assessment"–it has links to several excellent company sites as well as some individual tests you can try.

Emotional Intelligence quiz–http://www.utne.com/azEQ.tmpl–interactive quiz from the *Utne Reader*, Nov/Dec 1995 by Daniel Goleman.

Keirsey Temperament and Character Web Site–http://www.keirsey.com/.

Psycho-Geometrics–http://www.drsusan.net–a somewhat off-beat but interesting self-assessment tool. Scroll to the bottom of the page and click on the I.T. Serve button to start test.

PsychTests.com–http://www/psychtests.com/tests/index.html–demo versions are available for most tests–some tests require you to sign up.

SBA Women's Business Center site has an excellent page of resources for managers–a few of them also apply to self-assessment for individuals http://www.onlinewbc. gov/docs/manage/; see also *Developing Your Team Building Skills*–http://www. onlinewbc.gov/docs/manage/team.html.

BIBLIOGRAPHY

Agada, John (1998), "Profiling Librarians with the Myers-Briggs Type Indicator: Studies in Self Selection and Type Stability," *Education for Information* 16 no. 1 (March), 57-68.

Archer, Sarah Brick (2001), " 'Be All That You Can Be': Developing and Marketing Professionalism in Academic Reference Librarianship," *The Reference Librarian* no. 73, 351-360.

Argyle, Michael (1981), *Social Skills and Work*. London: Methuen.

Bryant, Susan (n.d.), *Think Outside the Box to Improve Your Cube Life*. [http:// content.monster.com/wlb/articles/attheoffice/cube].

Eckwright, Gail Z., Hoskisson, Tam, and Pollastro, Mike (1998), "Reference Etiquette: A Guide to Excruciatingly Correct Behavior," *American Libraries* 29, no. 5 (May), 42-45.

Eidson, Marshall (2000), "Using 'Emotional Intelligence' in the Reference Interview," *Colorado Libraries* 26, no. 2 (Summer), 8-10.

Flowers, Janet L. (2000), "Emotional Intelligence in the Workplace–Report from the 1999 Charleston Conference," *Library Collections, Acquisitions, and Technical Services* 24, no. 3 (Fall), 431-433.

Giesecke, Joan and McNeil, Beth (1999), "Core Competencies and the Learning Organization," *Library Administration & Management* 13, no. 3 (Summer), 158-166.

Goleman, Daniel (1998), *Working with Emotional Intelligence*. New York: Bantam Books.

Golian, Linda Marie (1999), "Thinking Style Preferences Among Academic Librarians: Practical Tips for Effective Work Relationships." In *Racing Toward Tomorrow: Proceedings of the Ninth National Conference of the Association of College & Research Libraries, April 8-11, 1999*. Chicago: The Association, 271-279.

Hoffman, Edward. (2002), *Psychological Testing at Work*. New York: McGraw-Hill.

Jones, Dixie A. (1997), "Plays Well with Others, or the Importance of Collegiality Within a Reference Unit," *The Reference Librarian* no. 59, 163-175.

Lee. Chris (1999), "Mean Streets and Rude Workplaces: The Death of Civility," *Training* 36 no. 7 (July), 24-30.

Levy, Philippa (1992), "Dimensions of Competence: Interpersonal Skills Development Within the LIS Curriculum," *Education for Information* 10, 87-103.

Levy, Philippa and Usherwood, Robert C. (1989), "Putting People First," *Library Association Record* 91 (September), 526, 529-530.

Manley, Will (1998), "Can't We All Get Along?" *American Libraries* 29 no. 11 (December), 104.

Marks, John (1996), "The American Uncivil Wars; How Crude, Rude and Obnoxious Behavior Has Replaced Good Manners and Why That Hurts Our Politics and Power," *U.S. News & World Report*, 120 no. 16 (April 22): 66-72.

Nofsinger, Mary M. (1999), "Training and Retraining Reference Professionals: Core Competencies for the 21st Century," *The Reference Librarian* no. 64, 9-19.

Pearson, Christine M., Andersson, Lynne M., and Porath, Christine L. (2000), "Assessing and Attacking Workplace Incivility," *Organizational Dynamics* 29 no. 2 (November), 123-137.

RASD Ad Hoc Committee on Behavioral Guidelines for Reference and Information Services (1996), *Guidelines for Behavioral Performance of Reference and Information Services Professionals* [http://www.ala.org/rusa/behavior.html], and reprinted in *RQ* 36 (Winter), 200-03.

Rosenstein, Linda L. (2000), "Emotional Intelligence in the Workplace–Report of a Program at ALA Midwinter 2000," *Library Collections, Acquisitions, and Technical Services* 24, no. 4 (Winter), 502-503.

Rosner, Bob (1998), *Working Wounded: Advice That Adds Insight to Injury*. New York: Warner Books.

Sherrer, Johannah (1996), "Thriving in Changing Times: Competencies for Today's Reference Librarians," *The Reference Librarian* no. 54, 11-20.

Special Library Association (October 1996), *Competencies for Special Librarians of the 21st Century* [http://www.sla.org/content/SLA/professional/meaning/competency.cfm].

Stueart, Robert D. (1989), "Human Relations in Library Education: Relationships Among Colleagues," *IFLA Journal* 15 no. 1, 44-49.

Terez, Tom (2002). *Civility at Work: 20 Ways to Build a Kinder Workplace* [http://www.betterworkplacenow.com/civilityart.html].

"Workplace Rudeness Is Common and Costly," *USA Today* 130, no. 2684 (May 2002): 9.

Building a Learning Culture
for the Common Good

Corinne Laverty
Melody Burton

SUMMARY. Librarians are well positioned to embrace the journey towards a learning culture; we have resources and we have incentive! Teetering on the edge of information technology, libraries are committed to continuous change for the benefit of our customers. To fulfill this promise, staff must keep pace with new technologies, products, and an increasing demand for new services in an environment with shrinking human resources. There is more to learn and less time in which to learn it. This paper describes a proactive, team-based approach used to create a learning culture in one library. Staff act as peer learners and teachers to educate themselves and each other about all aspects of their reference work such as approaches to service, orientation for new members, learning and evaluating new tools, and discussing the development of new services. The whole is greater than the sum–this dynamic, shared learning environment embraces diverse learning styles including discovery, discussion, demonstration, presentation, homework, questioning, and hands-on practice. Analysis of feedback from students and challenging questions at the reference desk grounded the experience and made it immediately relevant

Corinne Laverty (E-mail: lavertyc@post.queensu.ca) and Melody Burton (E-mail: burtonm@post.queensu.ca) are both Reference Librarians in a humanities and social sciences library at Stauffer Library, 101 Union Street, Queen's University, Kingston, Ontario, Canada K7L 5C4.

[Haworth co-indexing entry note]: "Building a Learning Culture for the Common Good." Laverty, Corinne, and Melody Burton. Co-published simultaneously in *The Reference Librarian* (The Haworth Information Press, an imprint of The Haworth Press, Inc.) No. 83/84, 2003, pp. 71-81; and: *Cooperative Reference: Social Interaction in the Workplace* (ed: Celia Hales Mabry) The Haworth Information Press, an imprint of The Haworth Press, Inc., 2003, pp. 71-81. Single or multiple copies of this article are available for a fee from The Haworth Document Delivery Service [1-800-HAWORTH, 9:00 a.m. - 5:00 p.m. (EST). E-mail address: docdelivery@haworthpress.com].

http://www.haworthpress.com/web/REF
Digital Object Identifier: 10.1300J120v40n83_07

and useful. This strategy furthers the goal of the learning organization where members share the responsibility of learning. The outcomes are an enriched collective knowledge and understanding, a sustainable model for continuous learning, social connectivity, and team experience. *[Article copies available for a fee from The Haworth Document Delivery Service: 1-800-HAWORTH. E-mail address: <docdelivery@haworthpress.com> Website: <http://www.HaworthPress.com> © 2003 by The Haworth Press, Inc. All rights reserved.]*

KEYWORDS. Learning culture, learning community, team-based learning, reference service, librarians' learning, learning organization

INTRODUCTION: THE NEED FOR LEARNING

There is more to learn and less time in which to learn it. In a comprehensive analysis of the world's entire sphere of data, researchers at the University of California at Berkeley (Lyman et al., 2000) estimate that the entire history of humanity accumulated 12 exabytes of information (1,000,000,000,000,000,000 bytes). Today 12 exabytes is produced every 2.5 years. While such calculations deal with publishing output, humanities and social sciences librarians feel this crunch as they attempt to keep pace with new electronic reference tools and simultaneously maintain competency with numerous print resources.

Queen's is a medium-sized university with a decentralized library. Reference service in the humanities and social sciences is provided by a core group of four librarians and augmented by contributions to reference desk hours by librarians from other units and two library assistants. In the summer of 2001, Queen's Libraries acquired several new electronic products or switched platforms for existing products. Additionally, several stable databases unveiled new interfaces. Recognizing that individual librarians were overwhelmed by the prospect of learning a plethora of new tools independently, humanities and social sciences librarians decided to devote a morning once or twice a month to learn these new or redesigned products in a teaching lab. The list of tools to explore was lengthy and immediately prompted the creation of a term-long schedule of topics. Individuals were assigned a database or subject grouping of databases to learn and present a "best practices" approach to their colleagues including relationships to print and other electronic resources, audience and evaluative comments. This was the beginning of our "learning sessions."

The simple division of work and the decision to share collectively in the learning of new databases were met with relief. Each librarian had been struggling to keep up with new products and an inability to do so resulted in a variety of unhealthy or unhelpful responses such as fear, insecurity, stress, ignorance, or avoidance of new databases.

TRANSFORMATION AND THE LEARNING ORGANIZATION

How are libraries tackling the learning necessary to keep pace with the explosion of information tools and technologies? The pressure for continual transformation has provided many libraries with an impetus to plan strategically for an evolution into "learning organizations." The emergence of this idea originates from the need for institutions to transform themselves internally in response to the advancement of the "information age" and the notion of the "learning society." A key feature of such an organization is its emphasis on developing a learning culture that supports both individual and collective learning. Donald Schön first described the notion that institutions must guide their own transformation through learning: "We must, in other words, become adept at learning. We must become able not only to transform our institutions, in response to changing situations and requirements; we must invent and develop institutions which are 'learning systems,' that is to say, systems capable of bringing about their own continuing transformation" (Schön, 1971).

Almost 20 years later, Peter Senge popularized the concept of the learning organization and proposed methods for achieving it in his work *The Fifth Discipline: The Art and Practice of the Learning Organization*. He outlines five "learning disciplines" that are at the core of the learning organization: personal mastery, mental models, shared vision, team learning, and systems thinking (Senge, 1990). Personal mastery relates to individual learning and is the key building block on which the learning organization is founded. Mental models describe how individuals think about their environment and how this influences their understanding and the actions they take. Shared vision identifies the need for group awareness of and commitment to a genuine goal. Teams, not individuals, are the fundamental learning units in contemporary organizations and their learning is accomplished through dialogue and collective thinking. The purpose of systems thinking is to understand relationships within the context of the whole enterprise rather than as isolated events or patterns.

Queen's Libraries began moving towards a team-based organizational structure in 1998. A prime motivation for this move was the need to address organizational illiteracy. During a review process it became clear that many library staff were knowledgeable only about their own departmental activities and few library staff understood or cared about the goals of the whole library system. Using the tenets of Senge's learning organization as a basis for this structure, a team-based organization promised to address some key deficiencies in our understanding of one another and promote an ongoing commitment to learning.

An organizational edict to become a team was met with optimism and skepticism. Within the Humanities and Social Sciences Reference Department, we adopted Senge's vocabulary and began to call ourselves a team, but in practice, we were typically a group of autonomous individuals who met regularly to discuss reference service, collections, and the latest addition to electronic holdings. In the summer of 2001, however, our learning needs became so great that our department had to address our existing learning strategies, abandon them, and adopt a shared approach to learning that could meet the escalating demands of our users. The convergence of becoming a team-based organization, adopting a learning organization philosophy and the compelling need to transform our learning behaviors became a natural point for change within our department. It also became a pivotal point in our history.

CREATING A LEARNING ENVIRONMENT

One would assume that librarians are exemplary learners, given their role as information mediators and their commitment to lifelong learning. Certainly librarians in Queen's Humanities and Social Sciences Reference Department demonstrated a commitment to learning when during a strategic planning session they voted "providing ongoing training for staff by working in a group together" as the second most popular initiative after "providing outreach to inform the university community about library services and resources" (Queen's University, 2001). Learning was formally acknowledged as a priority.

In what ways do learning initiatives play out within a reference unit in a single library? Librarians as adult learners need mechanisms to update continually their knowledge of new resources and technologies. They also need to consider how these resources complement existing tools and test strategies for their integration at the reference desk. Opportunities usually arise in the form of "training" sessions that are organized by administrators or opportunistically scheduled by vendors. A typical scenario is a demonstration or hands-on workshop where attention is given to technical operations such as search strategy and downloading options. A group of library staff who represent diverse user groups (e.g., Law, Science, Humanities, etc.) join together to learn about a new tool and how it works. Although these sessions provide a useful introduction, they neither address discipline-related applications nor provide a means to enrich the collective knowledge of the workforce. Without more in-depth analysis of the resource as it relates to specific areas of study or how it complements other tools, these sessions cannot provide a nurturing learning experience. Librarians need "know how," "know why" and "know who" when it comes to information tools. They must explore the content of new databases, test their applicability to areas of research, compare them to existing resources and understand their audience. Essential learning abilities travel the entire continuum of Bloom's learning skills taxonomy ranging from knowledge of factual information at the most basic level through comprehension, application, analysis, synthesis, to evaluation at the most complex level (Bloom, 1956). Each level is associated with an intellectual outcome and the type of questions associated with each category prompts critical thinking, especially in the higher levels. Table 1 matches the library learning questions we raised during our sessions to the learning categories expressed in Bloom's structure.

Movement through this learning hierarchy requires a learning environment not commonly found in the culture of most libraries. Learning can no longer be managed entirely as an independent activity where individuals are responsible for advancing their knowledge through formal courses or self-paced tutorials. Johnston and Hawke (2002) describe the new orientation in organizations toward building and maintaining a learning culture. In their investigation of the approaches used by six Australian organizations, they identify consistently successful strategies that promote movement towards a learning orientation:

- Use organizational pressures as an impetus to increase commitment to organizational learning. Pressures for change from the external environment should be examined for the learning opportunities they can instigate.
- Include learning initiatives that are more wide-ranging than formal training opportunities such as work-based components directly related to an individual's job activities where what is learned is directly linked to the work experience.

- Increase capacity of employees to contribute to decision-making.
- Foster a communicative work environment and the use of work relationships as a source of learning. Learning opportunities should be encouraged and supported by the organization, especially those involving collaborative work-based problems. Workers should share their learning and see one another as learning resources.
- Encourage an ethos of employee's accepting more responsibility for learning.

Libraries are well-positioned to adopt these strategies; change is constant in our environment and provides a commanding impetus for learning. Linking learning activities to real work tasks meshes well with the team-based initiatives in which staff join together to make decisions and direct learning enquiries. Our system-wide Information Services and Instruction Team, for example, is currently learning about virtual reference through reading, testing, attending conferences, asking questions, and contacting other institutions. They will use their learning as the basis for recommendations to the library system as a whole. Project work that emanates from internal teams fosters resident expertise where individuals and groups accept the responsibility for both learning and sharing their learning directly with colleagues and generally within the organization.

Another factor that contributes to successful learning experiences is taking into account the preferred learning strategies of the staff. Ways in which adults learn are described by Malcolm Knowles in his theory of andragogy (Knowles, 1984). Adults are self-directed learners who wish to be in charge of what they learn, how they learn, and when they learn. They are goal-oriented in that they become ready to learn when a specific need arises and are generally motivated to learn from within themselves rather than from external forces. Adults prefer a problem-centered orientation to learning that draws on real-life applications rather than hypothetical situations and draw on their own life experiences as a resource for learning.

Apart from the basic attributes of adult learners identified by Knowles, there are others that play an important part within a learning organization. Conner remarks that transfer of learning between employees is largely a function of the quality and strength of interpersonal relationships (Conner, 2002). This implies that even when learning is part of the daily fabric of institutional work, it is the social dimension of how staff perceive the knowledge of others that contributes to the development of a true learning culture. From this perspective, learning scenarios that

TABLE 1. Learning Questions Matched to Bloom's Taxonomy

Bloom's Learning Levels	Librarians' Learning Questions from Our Educational Sessions
Knowledge: the ability to recall factual information (list, define, describe, identify, show, label).	What kind of information is here? What time period is covered? How can this information be made accessible to students?
Comprehension: the lowest level of understanding where information can be restated, interpreted, compared, predicted (summarize, interpret, contrast, predict, differentiate, discuss, extend).	What is the content of this tool? From which sources is the information derived? How is this searched? In which sequence is this searched? What special features are available? What are the key concepts in this topic?
Application: the ability to apply knowledge in a specific situation (apply, demonstrate, complete, illustrate, examine, modify, relate, experiment, discover).	How does it relate to known subjects or assignments? How would a useful search query be expressed here? What are the possible research steps given a specific investigation question?
Analysis: the ability to break information into its component parts to reveal its organization, relationships, patterns (analyze, separate, order, explain, connect, classify, arrange, divide, compare, select, explain, infer).	What level of information is provided? What is the complexity of the content? How is this related to other information tools? How can students learn to use this? How do search results compare with other sources? Analyze search results to determine more effective search terms.
Synthesis: the ability to assemble component parts into a meaningful whole, use known ideas to create new ideas, generalize from facts, predict or draw conclusions (combine, integrate, modify, plan, create, invent, rewrite).	What is the role of this tool within the overall research strategy? What other pieces are missing? What needs to be added?
Evaluation: the ability to set standards by which to judge information, compare and discriminate between ideas, assess value, present a reasoned argument, verify evidence, recognize subjectivity (assess, rank, test, measure, recommend, judge, evaluate, explain, compare).	What is the accuracy and scope of sources included? How well does this address specific research needs? What content is missing? What are its limitations and deficiencies? What criteria can be articulated for evaluating sources?

isolate staff members, such as online tutorials or training for individuals outside the institution, are not as desirable as face-to-face instruction where relationships between peers can be forged. Cross states that research on the information environment of individuals indicates that work relationships have a significant impact for obtaining information, solving problems, and learning work-related activities (Cross, 2001). Knowledge of different people's area of expertise, for example, is a precursor for getting help with specific problems. Apart from knowing to whom one can turn, it is important that providing access to internal expertise is acknowledged within the organization as a means for learning.

In drawing on these learning principles, it is possible to aid the evolution of an organic learning environment that is shaped and created by its members. Learners should know why they are studying something and should be involved in the planning and evaluation of their instruction. Learners should be able to relate what is being studied to their personal and professional experiences. Instruction should be problem-centered and involve dialogue and knowledge construction. Learners will benefit from a scaffolding approach where more support is given in the early learning stages and it gradually declines until learners become self-reliant (Collis, 2002). In a constructive approach, teachers should see themselves as facilitators and co-learners. Vygotsky used "the zone of proximal development" (ZPD) to describe how collegial instructors can have a positive impact on the overall learning outcomes on their peers. The ZPD is " . . . the distance between the actual development level as determined by independent problem solving and the level of potential development as determined through problem solving under adult guidance or in collaboration with more capable peers" (Vygotsky, 1978). In other words, the ZPD is the difference between the quality of a learner's inquiry without assistance rather than with assistance. If peer interaction is to influence cognitive development, a collaborative learning environment is needed where individuals construct their own understanding through participation and group problem solving with others who are at different developmental levels. Successful learning strategies include sharing problem-solving methods for reference questions, modeling an approach to answering a question, or using a database after group input on key points, and taking turns as teacher. Teachers must bear in mind, however, that learners are individuals with different life experiences and learning preferences. Some adult learners will still prefer a traditional pedagogical approach to teaching and learning. Teachers should respect that, and at the same time gradually try to push learners away from their comfort zone in the direction of a deeper approach to learning.

FROM THEORY INTO PRACTICE

The educational theory described above can be detected in the learning sessions held by and for our team of humanities and social sciences reference staff. Examples of learning situations follow and reveal the tenets for creating a successful organizational learning culture: group

identification and commitment, shared common purpose and decision-making, reliance on one another, open communication, respect for
experience and knowledge of others, and contributing to learning experiences that are grounded in practice but focus on critical thinking skills.
In an early attempt to bring the group together, two librarians braved the
topic of approaches to reference service. This session opened the door
to a candid discussion of how individuals interact with library users,
subtleties of the reference interview, and sensitivities around how to
recognize and handle questions beyond an individual's capability. This
was the first step in building trust and a shared purpose with colleagues.
Members expressed alarm at the changing nature of reference questions; they take longer to answer, frequently require exploration of multiple sources, and users have great expectations of quick and accurate
answers. We were experiencing "techno-stress." Learning about new
resources was happening on the fly at the desk and we were learning by
the seat of our pants! The idea of depending on one another and collectively agreeing to learn together was born.

Initially the need for sessions was so great that individual librarians
took on the responsibility for learning a reference tool and imparting
an "insider's" evaluation of it. When a handful of nineteenth-century
literary and newspaper databases were available as a trial, the team felt
uncomfortable evaluating the databases and confessed their lack of
confidence with existing tools. The team's admission that competency
had lapsed helped the team bond and formed a common starting point
for learning. The session focused on print sources and electronic
sources, improving an overall understanding of what tools are available
and how they work together to provide coverage for this time period.
Since literature courses often require sources from the 1800s, approaches to searching materials by literary genre or for primary materials were illustrated. Linking tools to real reference problems greatly
contributed to the learning experience and enabled participants to carry
their inquiry well beyond the basic knowledge and comprehension
phases of questioning to higher level thinking skills.

The importance of applying learning and relating it to what we already
knew soon became obvious in our discussions. Therefore, to supplement learning sessions, a binder of "challenging questions" was collected at the reference desk so staff could record questions and potential
answers. Our group reviews these on an ongoing basis so that both successful and unsuccessful approaches are exchanged. We discovered
that sharing tactics on how to proceed when searches yield little or no

useful information was enlightening. Each of us has strategies for dealing with this but some are more productive than others.

In a large first-year undergraduate sociology class, two librarians assessed reference tools for their capacity to meet the needs of the class assignment. A series of workshops detailing an approach to the assignment was created and delivered for the students. The team received the assignment and devoted a meeting to strategies for the assignment and methods for teaching students at the reference desk. Ideas included how to dissect a null search set, identifying false matches, and how to discuss the hierarchy of sources with students at the desk.

One learning session was devoted to business sources. After a few false starts, the team was adamant that the approach to the session mirror the problem-based approach that students present at the reference desk. In other words, reference librarians wanted to approach the sources from the same vantage point as students and faculty, not from the point of view of how the collection is arranged but how it is used. Learning consequently stemmed from analyzing frequently-asked questions and the subject guide on the library website was changed to reflect this teaching method.

A current series of learning sessions on government documents abandons the familiar approach to the literature by genre (legislation, statistics) and jurisdiction (federal, international). Instead the sessions are a set of examples drawn from assignments that tackle the material in a thematic way, the same way in which students encounter the library and its resources. Sample topics include environmental pollution, women's reproductive rights and behaviors, youth and crime. This also provides the rich opportunity to understand how all humanities and social sciences tools might be used to address students' research needs. This requires a broad understanding of all reference tools and how they interrelate.

FROM LEARNING CULTURE TO LEARNING COMMUNITY

Learning organizations need to establish a culture of learning to sustain knowledge building from within. When learning is valued and supported in an organization the groundwork is laid for the development of learning teams or communities. It takes a community to establish common practices for learning and see themselves and each other as resources for learning. Learning experiences are richer because interaction encourages curiosity, potential, creativity, and offers new perspectives and opportunities for questioning. Shared responsibility for learning reduces the stress of independent study where individuals work alone or postpone their learning and tend not to communicate what they know. Learning together supports the process as an emotional as well as intellectual process; problem solving requires a revelation of feelings and attitudes, as well as ideas and questions. In observing others in the practice of learning, we also encourage new approaches to learning at the reference desk. In fact, we join our students in becoming part of the learning cycle that supports all of us.

REFERENCES

Bloom, Benjamin Samuel (1956). *Taxonomy of Educational Objectives: The Classification of Educational Goals*. New York: Longmans.

Collis, Betty, and Koos Winnips (2002)."Two Scenarios for Productive Learning Environments in the Workplace," *British Journal of Educational Technology* 33 (March): 133-148.

Conner, Marcia L., and James G. Clawson (2002). "Creating a Learning Culture." Paper presented at: Creating a Learning Culture: Strategy, Technology, and Practice. (University of Virginia). Available at http://www.darden.edu/batten/clc/Articles/clc.pdf.

Cross, Rob, Andrew Parker, Laurence Prusak, and Stephen P. Borgatti (2001). "Knowing What We Know: Supporting Knowledge Creation and Sharing in Social Networks," *Organizational Dynamics* 30 (November): 100-120.

Imel, Susan (1994). *Guidelines for Working with Adult Learners*. (ERIC Document Reproduction Service No.: ED377313) Johnston, Robyn, and Geof Hawke (2002). *Case Studies of Organisations with Established Learning Cultures*. Leabrook: National Centre for Vocational Education Research. Available at http://www.ncver.edu.au.

Knowles, Malcolm S. (1984). *Andragogy in Action: Applying Modern Principles of Adult Learning*. San Francisco: Jossey-Bass.

Libutti, Patricia. O'Brien (Ed.) (1999). *Librarians as Learners, Librarians as Teachers: The Diffusion of Internet Expertise in the Academic Library*. Chicago: Association of College and Research Libraries.

Lyman, Peter, and Hal R. Varian (2000). School of Information Management and Systems at the University of California at Berkeley. "How Much Information?" Available at http://www.sims.berkeley.edu/research/projects/how-much-info/.

Queen's University. Humanities and Social Sciences Reference Department (2001). "Strategic Initiative Setting Session." Working paper. Queen's University, Kingston Ontario, Canada.

Schön, Donald A. (1971). *Beyond the Stable State: Public and Private Learning in a Changing Society*. London: Temple Smith.

Senge, Peter. M. (1990). *The Fifth Discipline: The Art and Practice of the Learning Organization*. New York: Doubleday/Currency.

Vygotsky, Lev Semenovich (1978). *Mind in Society: The Development of Higher Psychological Processes*. Cambridge, MA: Harvard University Press.

WORKING WITHIN THE LIBRARY: PRACTICALITIES

Crossing Three Bridges: Linking Librarianship and Teaching Across the P-16 Educational Continuum

Tracy L. Hull

Natalia Taylor

SUMMARY. Georgia State University Library's Education and Communication liaisons teamed up to teach a graduate course on the selection and use of reference resources for the College of Education's Library Media Technology Program. The collaboration between these two librarians can serve as a model for collaboration on three levels: collaboration between two librarians as co-teachers; collaboration be-

Tracy L. Hull is Head of Information Services, W. W. Hagerty Library, Drexel University, Philadelphia, PA 19104 (E-mail: tlh29@drexel.edu). At the time this was written, she was Department Head of Liaison and Research Services, Pullen Library, Georgia State University, Atlanta, GA. Natalia Taylor is Education Liaison Librarian, Pullen Library, Georgia State University, 100 Decatur Street, SE, Atlanta, GA 30303 (E-mail: natalia@gsu.edu).

[Haworth co-indexing entry note]: "Crossing Three Bridges: Linking Librarianship and Teaching Across the P-16 Educational Continuum." Hull, Tracy L., and Natalia Taylor. Co-published simultaneously in *The Reference Librarian* (The Haworth Information Press, an imprint of The Haworth Press, Inc.) No. 83/84, 2003, pp. 83-96; and: *Cooperative Reference: Social Interaction in the Workplace* (ed: Celia Hales Mabry) The Haworth Information Press, an imprint of The Haworth Press, Inc., 2003, pp. 83-96. Single or multiple copies of this article are available for a fee from The Haworth Document Delivery Service [1-800-HAWORTH, 9:00 a.m. - 5:00 p.m. (EST). E-mail address: docdelivery@haworthpress.com].

http://www.haworthpress.com/web/REF
Digital Object Identifier: 10.1300J120v40n83_08

tween university librarians and academic department faculty; and, finally, "collaboration across work places" between academic librarians and school media specialists in P-12 settings. Unique challenges, benefits, and possibilities for this type of collaborative effort are examined. *[Article copies available for a fee from The Haworth Document Delivery Service: 1-800-HAWORTH. E-mail address: <docdelivery@haworthpress.com> Website: <http://www.HaworthPress.com> © 2003 by The Haworth Press, Inc. All rights reserved.]*

KEYWORDS. Collaboration, P-16, media specialists, reference, instruction, college, university

INTRODUCTION

Those outside our profession often think of librarianship as an isolated and lonely job. As many of us know, the reality is quite different. The library profession revolves around cooperation, group work, and partnership. This article will discuss the collaboration of two academic librarians in the teaching of a core class for the Library Media Technology (MLM) program at Georgia State University. We will explain its significance as a model for collaboration on three levels: collaboration between two librarians as co-teachers; collaboration between university librarians and academic department faculty resulting in a strengthening of the liaison model; and most importantly, "collaboration across work places" between academic librarians and school media specialists in P-12 settings.

LITERATURE REVIEW

As most academic librarians know and as indicated in the literature, recent high school graduates entering college often have a significant deficiency in their research knowledge and information literacy skills. Partnerships have been developing between high schools and university libraries for a number of years, as professionals from both institutions strive to remedy this problem. Many of these efforts have been quite successful; but given the pervasiveness of the knowledge gap, there needs to be a more systematic effort in both the fields of education and librarianship to better prepare students for college-level research. The importance of devoting attention and resources to this issue only grows more apparent as the amount of accessible information continues to increase rapidly.

A variety of collaborative efforts across the academic continuum are cited in the literature, although the level of involvement between institutions varies considerably. Given that high school libraries frequently have limited resources, collaboration seems only logical. For universities, on the other hand, the most cited benefit in forming collaborative partnerships with P-12 institutions is to increase recruitment to the university or to the profession.

Early partnership projects, such as the collaboration in the early 1990s between University of California at Davis and Davis Senior High School, were driven by a lack of computer resources within the public school (Meizel, 1992). Due to public school budget cuts, caused by the poor economy at the time, the Davis Senior High School found itself with outdated print resources and with inadequate technological resources. At first, the partnership with UC Davis focused on improving the computer studies curriculum; but the collaborative effort soon expanded to provide high school students with the research skills they would need when they reached college.

Whereas lack of computers was the primary problem in the early '90s, the main issue today is students' lack of proficiency in using technological resources to access relevant information. What prospective college students need, then, is not simply more computers, but systematic instruction on the appropriate use and evaluation of information retrieved through these channels. Back in the years of the UC-Davis project, one of the daunting tasks facing high school students, according to Meizel (1992), was learning how to deal with the overabundance of materials available on the Internet. Students were overwhelmed by the plethora of documents and resources that they encountered in the virtual domain, finding it difficult to narrow their searches. With the rapid increase in the availability of information via the Web, this problem has only grown worse.

Numerous other collaborative efforts are cited in the literature. The highly successful University of Nebraska High School Users Program, which began in 1980, focused on bringing high school students up to speed, by supplying them with basic research skills and allowing them to borrow materials (Pearson and McNeil, 2002). Along similar lines, The University of Wisconsin-Madison College Library collaborated with school groups in the early 1990s (Jesudason, 1993). This effort relied principally on self-instructional tours and packets.

In 1995, the Brooklyn College Library and two New York City high schools entered into the privately funded Cooperative Library Project, which provided bibliographic instruction not only to the students, but also to their teachers and school librarians (Evans, 1997). This program underscored the differences in the students' research knowledge at the two levels (i.e., high school and college) and identified areas of deficiency in both teachers and librarians. The high school librarians needed to sharpen their skills in using resources they did not have in their own libraries, while the teachers had to become more familiar with current resources and research methodologies at the college level.

While many programs involving cooperation between colleges and secondary schools are still active, many are abandoned after only a few years, usually because they are perceived as not achieving their potential (Simon, 1992). This is unfortunate, considering the exigency for producing information literate students. With the Internet and access to information expanding rapidly, high school students are developing their own, often inefficient or even misguided, methods of finding information. Collaborative efforts between schools and university libraries can help instill in these young people the necessary skill sets to support lifelong learning.

Cahoy, who has made the transition from being a school library media specialist to an information literacy librarian at a university library, notes that there are new initiatives forming with the P-16 movement that highlight aligning standards at all levels (Cahoy, 2002). Progress has been made with the publications of information literacy standards by not only the American Association of School Librarians (AASL) and the Association for Educational Communications and Technology (AECT), in 1998, but also the Association of College and Research Libraries (ACRL), in 2000. While these two sets of standards differ–the former defining the underlying concept of what it means to be information literate and the latter being more skills focused–Cahoy points out that the ACRL standards indicate that they should be viewed as a continuation of the AASL/AECT standards.

Commentators argue that such high standards of information literacy cannot happen without strong partnerships between academic librarians and school library media specialists (Cahoy, 2002). And these partnerships, in turn, will not develop unless teachers and librarians share a common objective, one that is fully supported by both school and university administration (Simon, 1992).

The authors of this article have had the opportunity to teach a course in Georgia State University's Library Media Technology Program which brought them in contact with future school library media specialists, many of whom have been teachers. The interaction in the classroom brought to light the strong need for collaborative efforts between secondary schools and universities to address deficiencies in college-bound students' research skills. The collaborative effort at Georgia State University is only a small beginning, but perhaps can serve as a base for more far-reaching efforts to help metro-Atlanta area schools address this pressing issue.

CONTEXT: GEORGIA STATE UNIVERSITY

Georgia State University is the second largest university in the state of Georgia with an enrollment of approximately 27,000 students representing all states and over 140 countries. The campus is in the heart of downtown Atlanta. It is located a few blocks from the state capital building, Underground Atlanta, and the central mass transit station for the city (Five Points MARTA).

In the past, this university was widely known as a commuter campus. Many of the students enrolled were older, held full-time jobs, and were seeking a first Bachelors degree. In recent years, this trend has changed. The university has attracted more traditional college students. The Fall 2002 enrollment was a record high. Many of these students are from the metro area and can easily commute to school; but with the addition of the 1996 "Olympic Village," which was converted into dormitories for the university, and the completion of married student loft apartments in August 2002, the university is enrolling more students in general, and more "traditional" college-aged students.

GSU has six colleges: College of Arts & Sciences, College of Education, Andrew Young School of Policy Studies, College of Health and Human Sciences, Robinson College of Business, and the College of Law. Within these colleges there are 52 undergraduate and graduate degree programs encompassing over 250 fields of study. The racial and ethnic diversity of the campus reflects the Atlanta metropolitan area and the campus is lively and brimming with activity during the week.

CONTEXT: THE LIBRARY

William Russell Pullen Library is located at the heart of the campus and serves as the main library on campus. Pullen Library also has a small branch library at the satellite Alpharetta Campus. Two additional libraries, which are not linked to Pullen Library, yet serve as additional resources for students on campus, are the College of Law Library and the College of Education's Information Technology Center (ITC). Both of those libraries are fairly small and subject specific. In the case of the ITC, this resource center focuses primarily on educational technology, software, and curriculum materials.

Pullen Library's collections consist of more than 1.3 million volumes, approximately 5,000 serial titles, 850,000 government documents, and over 12,000 media titles. There are roughly 135 people currently employed at Pullen, 40 of whom are professional librarians. A majority of those librarians serve as liaison librarians to the university's academic departments.

The liaison model was initiated in 1998. Originally the library operated with the traditional four or five bibliographers who selected items for the general areas of humanities, social sciences, sciences, etc. With the liaison model, there was a push to hire more librarians who could specialize in the various subject areas represented by the University's degree programs. The current structure consists of twenty librarians who collect for their specialized subject areas. Most liaisons are responsible for two or three subject areas.

In addition to collection development for specialized subject areas, the liaisons participate in library instruction for their areas and general reference, as well as act as advocates for their departments. With the outreach work that the liaisons do with their departments, the librarians gain a better understanding of the library resources essential for those subject areas, at the same time that the academic faculty learn what the library has to offer and what additional support the library needs from the university. The liaisons work in subject clusters, connecting back to the original subject bibliographer model, to enable collaborative collection development in an increasingly interdisciplinary academic environment.

CONTEXT: LIBRARY MEDIA TECHNOLOGY PROGRAM

The Library Media Technology Program is a graduate program based in the College of Education's Department of Middle Secondary Education and Instructional Technology (MSIT) at Georgia State University. It prepares students to serve as library media specialists and information technologists in P-12 school environments. The program is not ALA accredited. The program began in 1973, offering the Masters of Library Media (MLM). There are currently full programs running at both the downtown campus and the satellite Alpharetta campus of GSU. There are approximately seventy Master's students with an additional twenty-two who are part of a unique cohort in Gwinnett County as the result of a special partnership between the College of Education and that county's Department of Education.

In addition to the Master's students, there are currently ten Ed.S. students and six Ph.D. students in Instructional Technology who are specializing in librarianship. The Master's students who enter the program without already having attained a teaching certification must take the course EXC 2010: Exceptional Children and Instruction, in addition to their MLM courses. All students must pass the Library Media Specialist area of the Praxis II test before receiving the MLM degree.

The Master's in Library Media Technology consists of 36 semester hours (12 courses). There are nine core courses and three additional courses chosen from eight options. The core courses range from Selection and Use of Reference Sources (ELMT 7130), the course taught by the authors, two Pullen Library librarians, to The Psychology of Learning and Learners. Three additional courses are chosen from three basic areas: Pedagogy and Social and Cultural Foundations of Education; Research Methods; and Instructional Technology.

OUR INVOLVEMENT

Our involvement with the course ELMT 7130 was due to two main factors. The first factor was that the MLM program was experiencing an unexpectedly low number of teaching faculty for the summer 2002 session due to unforeseen and unavoidable consequences. The second factor was that the Education Liaison Librarian had developed a relationship with the department and program dating back to 2000, and both parties had repeatedly mentioned the possibility of exploring avenues for collaboration. Because the Education Liaison had a background in the field of education, as well as experience as a librarian, the MLM program faculty believed that she would be able to offer insight into the subject matter. When presented with this opportunity, the Education Liaison turned to the Communication Liaison who had more years of experience with reference and who also had been the first-year instruction coordinator at Duke University.

Collaborating with another librarian was beneficial because it allowed for the natural sharing of ideas, which happens when co-teaching. Moreover, since neither librarian had taught a graduate level 3-credit hour course, it only made sense to divide the duties between them, since teaching the course alone could be an overwhelming experience. The partnership between the Education and the Communication Liaison Librarians helped win over the Library and College of Education administration, largely due to the fact that both the education and the media perspectives would be represented. Having the support of both the College of Education and Pullen Library administrations was of utmost importance. Without the support of these parties, the librarians would never have been able to successfully teach the course. The University Librarian has encouraged librarians to teach when the opportunity arises as a way of integrating the library more visibly into university affairs. As Simon (1992) has clearly argued, support from the relevant administrative units is crucial for a successful collaborative effort.

OUR EXPERIENCES WITH ELMT 7130

Our involvement with the course from the beginning involved collaboration and extensive communication with the faculty within the program. The head of the MLM program shared her previous resources with us and helped us to formulate our ideas regarding the progression and content of the course. We relied on this input and collaboration, and combined it with our own professional experiences and our memory of the reference courses we had each had during our MLS training. Both of us had greatly enjoyed our reference courses during our MLS studies, and had benefited from these courses considerably. Consequently, we referred often to our experiences as students in order to inform our teaching practices.

COURSE CONTENT

The course was very interactive. With the team teaching structure, we were able to take on different topics of discussion according to our levels of interest and expertise. Frequently, we would have a brief lecture followed by discussion of the topic and readings, and issues encountered while completing the reference assignments. The texts utilized for the course were Bopp and Smith's *Reference and Informa-tion Services: An Introduction* and Katz's *Introduction to Reference Work*. These texts complimented each other and provided thorough coverage of the course content.

ASSIGNMENTS

Six of the assignments were the standard "reference assignments" in which students become familiar with different types of resources by an-swering typical reference questions. The students were provided with a bibliography of the different types of resources in which the answers could be found.

In addition to the reference assignments, the students were required to complete four other assignments. One was an observation and write up of the reference interview interaction as observed at a local library reference desk. The second assignment required them to develop a spe-cialized reference collection and present a bibliography that included summaries, justification, pricing, and reviews of resources that fit their chosen topic and grade levels. Another assignment required them to compare two similar reference resources, either print or electronic. Finally, the last assignment was a group project requiring the students to conduct a library instruction session. By providing this variety of as-signments, we conveyed both the practical and more nuanced or cre-ative aspects of reference work.

LESSONS LEARNED

As with any first endeavor, teaching the MLM course provided the instructors with information that would inform our execution of the course in the future. We had chosen to focus on print resources early in the course, and then cover the electronic resources when addressing in-dexes and abstracting resources. We learned that it would have been helpful to incorporate the electronic resources earlier in the course, as well as provide a more comprehensive introduction to the Pullen Li-brary System and e-resources early on.

Another lesson learned was that the students wanted as much struc-ture as possible, both in the lectures and the assignments. This seems to be the case with College of Education students in general, and could be due to a variety of factors, which would require several additional articles to explore. We also learned that the workload should be as evenly distributed throughout the course as possible. Because the course was taught in the summer session, which is less than half as long as a regular session, time compression was a significant factor in the course. We scheduled the time-intensive reference question assignments early in the course, so that students could complete them before assignments for their other courses became due. These questions tended to require a great deal more patience than the evaluation, selection, and instruction assignments, which came later in the course. Having to deal with such demanding tasks right off the bat was debilitating for some of the students' self-confidence, as they had not had a chance to prove their competence, to themselves as well as to the instructors, through successful completion of less demanding assignments. Varying the types of assignments would have benefited the students' morale by alternating between more and less difficult tasks.

We also learned that most of the students needed a thorough introduction to the resources in class lectures prior to searching them for their reference assignments. Due to the fact that we, the instructors, learn best by doing, we mistakenly assumed that the students would, like ourselves, not prefer a thorough introduction, but would rather prefer to jump right into the resources and then find out more details later. Students expressed unease with this process, and said that a thorough description of each resource prior to doing assignments would be much appreciated.

OBSERVATIONS AND OUTCOMES

Students were very eager to learn the material. Often after class, students would stay to talk with us and mine us for information until we had to, figuratively, push them away so we could return to our work. The students came to the class representing an array of experiences. We had several students in the class who were already teachers in the classroom. On the other hand, we had a number of students who had never set foot in a classroom as a teacher. An interesting phenomenon was that we had several students who were currently working at Atlanta-based CNN. They saw the MLM degree as a way to continue pursuing their interest in media and information while also "making a difference" in the future generation. They saw the MLM degree and a future in school media technology as a viable alternative to their current careers. We also had other students who had completed full careers in other areas and were looking for a complete change of pace. They were drawn to school media technology for a variety of reasons.

The students who came to the class with teaching backgrounds provided a very useful context for the course material. While we could bring our experiences of working with diverse populations in a large urban research institution, these students provided input regarding the school context that was invaluable. We were able to learn from those who had taught, and the interaction highlighted some of the differences in research knowledge–much like the experience in the Cooperative Library Project at Brooklyn College (Evans, 1997).

Student reactions to the course were overall quite positive. We received high evaluation ratings from the students, which was particularly comforting given that this was the first time we had taught the course. The students had very positive reactions to the idea of having practitioners teach the course. They also appreciated the team teaching model and felt that the different backgrounds and teaching styles of the instructors was beneficial and added a sense of variety. Several students commented that this had been their "favorite" course in the program, which was a real surprise since we had heard from students within the department that it was the course that students often dreaded and feared the most. An unexpected outcome was that several students expressed interest in academic librarianship and asked about requirements and ALA-accredited programs which would allow them to go into a university setting.

One of the ELMT 7130 students began serving as a graduate assistant at the Pullen Library reference desk. This unexpected outcome was invaluable as she came to the position with extensive training in the materials available at the Pullen Library. There was also an increased recognition of librarians as teachers at the university level due to our involvement with the program and course. Another positive outcome was a sense of commitment between the library and the MLM program. We shared our materials and experiences with the instructor who taught the course in the fall semester and she considered this input invaluable.

A substantial outcome of our collaborative teaching experience was the creation of a mentoring environment in the workplace. Students have dropped by the library to share their experiences with us and to ask us for advice regarding their other MLM courses or, for those who have graduated, their new school environments. We are currently in the process of making arrangements with those students who have completed the program to make site visits to their schools. This will serve two purposes. It will not only provide support for them at their posts, but will also help inform us of the situation of school media specialists in the schools and ways in which we, as academic librarians, might increase our partnership between the university and the school system.

Another positive outcome has been a better local understanding, on both sides of the P-16 continuum, of the library resources that are available for school-aged children. This includes not only the media and reference resources that can be utilized by middle and high school students, but also the juvenile collection the library maintains, as well as the school-aged appropriate resources in GALILEO, Georgia's networked system of databases.

One of the most beneficial outcomes of this collaboration has been the increased awareness on the part of the future media specialists of the importance of information literacy. By the end of the course, the students understood that there are fundamental information literacy skills we expect incoming university freshmen to have, and that the building blocks for these skills must be developed from the very beginning of the P-12 process with the help of school library media specialists. The collaboration helped bridge the gap that has been created between the information literacy competencies and language at the college and university level, on the one hand, and the research skills currently being taught at most P-12 schools, on the other.

Other positive outcomes have included increased recognition of the Education Liaison within the MSIT department. She achieved further name recognition, and was perceived as more of a colleague than a completely separate entity "over there in the library," as was the case before. She noted that she received requests for bibliographic instruction sessions from others in the department who had not previously made such contact with her. In addition, the department asked her to serve on a search committee for the program. In short, there was a greater sense of shared commitment and purpose.

BUILDING BRIDGES

Based on our experiences, and seeing how enthusiastic these students were, we became very interested in determining how we could reach out as academic librarians to the schools in the metropolitan Atlanta area. Many of our students were teachers, yet had very little knowledge of information literacy or how to locate resources and do library research. When first-year students come to GSU, we often note this gap in their training. They lack the sophisticated research skills needed for college level research papers. This is not a problem that is new to the profession of academic librarianship. Many academic librarians are faced with this problem every fall when the new freshman class arrives on campus. This pervasive experience raises the question, what collaborative efforts are underway and in what additional ways can academic librarians and school library media specialists bridge this knowledge gap? Many schools that offer library media specialist programs, along with library schools, often offer summer institutes, and some academic libraries reach out to their local community high schools to help college-bound students acquire these skills, but these are only beginning steps. Such efforts, though certainly laudable, are small in comparison to the number of students and schools that are not so fortunate to have this contact with academic librarians.

In an age when information literacy is becoming a necessary set of skills, there needs to be a broader and more systematic effort to bridge the gap between academic and P-12 institutions. At the 2002 Georgia Council of Media Organizations (GaCOMO) conference, we presented a preliminary version of this article and spent time describing our experiences and brainstorming about possible collaborative avenues with the attendees. Many agreed that a larger collaborative effort is overdue. One attendee recommended statewide or even national competencies that schools should be required to teach, and that students should have to prove proficiency in prior to graduation.

Other librarians in attendance suggested more outreach programs at local colleges and universities, which would allow academic librarians to work with the school library media specialists to identify aspects of research about which many college-bound students are ignorant. Through outreach programs like this one, the academic librarian could teach information literacy sessions to the college-bound students or collaborate with the school library media specialist to help devise avenues to teach these skill sets to the students.

While collaboration across institutions and work place environments can lead to great benefits for all involved, it can also be quite time consuming and require skills that most academic librarians or school media specialists do not normally have. In addition to eliciting support and encouragement from the administrative units involved, interpersonal skills, such as conflict-resolution and mediation, should be fostered in the participants. The academic and P-12 environments cultivate vastly different workplace cultures, and additional sensitivity and awareness will be necessary to work together effectively. As both Jesudason (1993) and Simon (1992) have pointed out, without intentional planning and clarity about communication, organizational objectives, and collaborative structures, these types of linkages may have limited endurance and success.

CONCLUSION

While there are many challenges to collaboration between P-12 and university libraries in an urban environment, such as that served by GSU, this type of cooperation ultimately benefits the university. By collaborating to help students in P-12 develop their library, research, and information literacy skills, library media specialists and university librarians can help students enter the university more prepared for academic success. This will reduce the wear and tear on academic librarians and instructors who work with first-year students. In addition, it will lead to greater retention, as students will be less frustrated and overwhelmed by the transition to higher education. Such efforts might possibly even increase interest in the librarian profession among the younger population: something that is desperately needed as we enter a crisis of recruitment in our profession. And finally, the collaboration can lead to a more enriched academic environment for all at the university and those in the immediate urban environment.

REFERENCES

Bopp, R. E. and Smith, L. C. (eds.) (2001), *Reference and Information Services: An Introduction* (3rd ed.). Englewood, CO: Libraries Unlimited.

Cahoy, E. S. (2002), "Will Your Students Be Ready for College? Connecting K-12 and College Standards for Information Literacy," *Knowledge Quest*, 30 (4), 12-15.

Evans, B. (1997), "Building Bridges Between New York City Public High Schools and a College: The Cooperative Library Project," *Research Strategies*, 15 (2), 89-99.

Jesudason, M. (1993), "Academic Libraries and Outreach Services Through Precollege Programs: A Proactive Collaboration," *RSR: Reference Services Review*, 21 (4), 29-36+.

Katz, W.A. (2002), *Introduction to Reference Work* (8th ed.). New York: McGraw Hill.

Meizel, J. (1992), "High School Education and the Internet: The Davis Senior High School Experience," *Resource Sharing & Information Networks*, 8 (1), 127-40.

Pearson, D. and McNeil, B. (2002), "From High School Users College Students Grow: Providing Academic Library Research Opportunities to High School Students," *Knowledge Quest*, 30 (4), 24-28.

Simon, M. (1992), "Forging New Organizational and Communications Structures: The College Library School Library Partnership," *Library Administration & Management*, 6 (1), 36-40.

Cooperative Reference Desk Scheduling and Its Effects on Professional Collegiality

Valery King

SUMMARY. Since 1995, reference staff at Oregon State University's Valley Library have engaged in a process of cooperative reference desk scheduling. The system was originally adopted to allow staff to have more influence in tailoring desk hours to their individual work schedules, but the department discovered that it also encourages and reinforces a climate of cooperation and collegiality among the reference staff. This paper describes the creation of the system and examines the reasoning behind it, the steps taken to implement it, and how it continues to evolve in an ever-changing library environment. Also examined is how this system has influenced other work done in the Reference and Instruction Department beyond the reference desk, and how it might be adapted and applied for use in other tasks in the future. *[Article copies available for a fee from The Haworth Document Delivery Service: 1-800-HAWORTH. E-mail address: <docdelivery@haworthpress.com> Website: <http://www.HaworthPress.com> © 2003 by The Haworth Press, Inc. All rights reserved.]*

KEYWORDS. Reference desk, scheduling, collegiality, cooperation

Valery King is Reference Librarian, The Valley Library, Oregon State University, 121 The Valley Library, Corvallis, OR 97331-4501 (E-mail: valery.king@orst.edu).

[Haworth co-indexing entry note]: "Cooperative Reference Desk Scheduling and Its Effects on Professional Collegiality." King, Valery. Co-published simultaneously in *The Reference Librarian* (The Haworth Information Press, an imprint of The Haworth Press, Inc.) No. 83/84, 2003, pp. 97-118; and: *Cooperative Reference: Social Interaction in the Workplace* (ed: Celia Hales Mabry) The Haworth Information Press, an imprint of The Haworth Press, Inc., 2003, pp. 97-118. Single or multiple copies of this article are available for a fee from The Haworth Document Delivery Service [1-800-HAWORTH, 9:00 a.m. - 5:00 p.m. (EST). E-mail address: docdelivery@haworthpress.com].

http://www.haworthpress.com/web/REF
Digital Object Identifier: 10.1300J120v40n83_09

How many librarians does it take to schedule a reference desk? The answer at Oregon State University's Valley Library is: all of them.

Through a unique group scheduling system, the reference staff at the main library (called the Valley Library) create their own desk schedules, and the system has been working since 1995. One of the forces driving the development of this system was the library's experimentation with team-based management in the 1990s, which created in the staff a climate of cooperation, an increase in collegiality, and a desire to take ownership of their day-to-day work. The Reference and Instruction Department makes the procedure work for them with the flexibility that's been built in, and they have discovered that it enhances their cooperation in other work done in the department.

LITERATURE SEARCH

Despite the fact that all libraries with reference desks go through some kind of process to schedule workers at that desk, there is surprisingly little to be found in the literature concerning it. Most books and articles, when they mention scheduling at all, include it under "staffing" and limit their discussions to hours covered and to the number and status of desk staff (Dennison, 1999). They are more interested in the result, rather than the process. Neville (1982) does at least acknowledge the importance of scheduling. "Although scheduling appears to be a rather minor matter and perhaps better included with staffing," she states, "my experience indicates that it can be a hot potato in the day-to-day affairs of a reference service."

Procedure is given more attention in articles concerning the use of computer programs to create schedules, primarily in relation to making the software program function (Cornick and Owen, 1988; deHaas, 1983). The most substantive article on reference desk scheduling is by Stelk and Lu (1997) which discusses the philosophical issues and human elements involved in reference desk scheduling.

DEVELOPING A NEW SYSTEM

The methods of reference service delivery have gone through major changes over the past two decades at OSU, and the methods for scheduling that delivery have had to adapt. The path to the current method of group self-scheduling at Oregon State University's main library began several years before the actual change was made.

The Valley Library is a six-story building, the only library on a campus of approximately 15,000 students. For many years there were three reference service points located on separate floors, each with a certain amount of autonomy: Science Reference, Social Science/Humanities Reference, and Government Documents. In 1988 two of these points, the Science and the Social Science/Humanities desks, were combined into one reference point on the main floor under a single department head (Butcher and Kinch, 1990). With the reorganization, a larger pool of reference personnel had to be scheduled for a single desk; previously, the two division heads scheduled smaller numbers of people for fewer hours at two separate desks. Scheduling the combined group of 18 librarians and six classified staff was assigned to the newly-named Assistant Head of Reference.

THE SKILLS OF A SCHEDULER

The task of scheduling this large number of staff at a reference desk in a busy academic setting is daunting. The responsibilities and skills required of a scheduler are outlined by Stelk and Lu (1997) and are complex and demanding: impartiality, consistency, flexibility, collegiality, diplomacy, devotion. According to them, the successful scheduler appears to need all the skills of a diplomat, a psychologist, a psychic, and a saint. For example, she is expected to know or discover:

- Shift preferences, vacation periods, and potential conflicts involving committee assignments, meetings, bibliographic instruction duties, and other activities.
- Knowledge of individuals' circumstances and obligations.

Some of this can be included on a pre-scheduling form, but when you have 24 people to schedule this creates a tremendous amount of paperwork.

OSU's PROCESS

The newly-combined main reference desk at OSU provided service for 77 hours each week including evenings and weekends. With double-scheduling and "backup" coverage for the busiest times there was a minimum of 116 service hours to fill per week. Once the Head of Reference and Assistant Head of Reference negotiated the number of hours each staff member would work at the desk per week, since not all staff worked "full time" desk hours, the Assistant Head asked the staff for their shift preferences (1st choice, 2nd choice, and "impossible"). She would then build a schedule taking these into account, as is done in most reference departments. In addition, she was directed to pair a science subject specialist with a social science/humanities subject specialist. The pairing was a good idea but it took the assistant many hours to produce a schedule adjusting for this as well as everything else a scheduler needs to keep in mind. And it was quickly apparent that with this larger group " . . . the scheduling process is even more complicated and time-consuming because with more staff involved, the problems of scheduling are compounded" (Stelk & Lu, 1997).

Purchase of scheduling software was briefly considered, but discarded. At the time there was nothing available that would adequately replace the manual preparation of the schedule. Money was also something of a concern, and at that time the few programs that were available were quite expensive. Other major drawbacks are that "scheduling software is not able to monitor the daily operation of a reference desk, or find a substitute when an emergency occurs; nor is it able to settle scheduling conflicts. Human efforts in this area are indispensable" (Stelk & Lu, 1997). The desk scheduler would therefore still need to play a significant role, even in an institution using software to create schedules. With even the best software, one person would still be making all the scheduling decisions despite worker input.

With so many other duties demanding the Assistant Head's time, the many hours needed to create a satisfactory schedule each term became untenable. A new way of creating a desk schedule was needed.

DEVELOPMENT OF THE GROUP SCHEDULING CONCEPT

Staff at the OSU libraries had learned to be adaptable and open to change, individually and as a group. Since 1989 OSU had experimented with Total Quality Management and other team-based management systems, and the result was a highly cooperative and team-oriented staff culture. (Butcher, 1993 and 1997; Davidson and Rusk, 1996). The library administration strongly support the view that staff are more effective and efficient "when they have direct responsibility for managing their day-to-day work" (Butcher, 1997). Staff have had a lot of practice in operating as a group, and have developed a great deal of professional pride and interest in working together to provide a high quality reference service to patrons. Everyone recognized that the achievements of an organization are "the result of the combined efforts of each individual in the organization working toward common objectives" (Stelk & Lu, 1997). With the extensive training all staff had received in team-based management, and their experience with forming management teams, they felt they had all the tools and training necessary to bring about this cooperative venture. This team training helped to create a climate of professionals willing–and wanting–to manage themselves and their work.

A group of classified staff and librarians on the Reference Center Management Team (RCMT) worked together on this plan. "This was vital in coming up with a process that worked," according to one member of the team. "I think having a group focus on the needs of the desk was the key to our success as far as scheduling goes. There was a lot of support for the process and much involvement from everyone. . . . everyone on RCMT at the time thought the desk was important enough to justify the hands-on effort."

The time was right for the idea of the staff scheduling themselves to be proposed. The department was willing to try this, even though traditionally "reference librarians are reluctant to take on managerial duties or become reference managers, and justifiably so. . . . They want someone else to solve the nitty-gritty problems . . . so that they can get on with what they do best" (King, 1987).

With the realization that, to a great extent, desk scheduling can be viewed as a collective responsibility and shared decision making (Stelk & Lu, 1997), a workgroup within the Reference Center Management Team came up with a self-scheduling concept and developed it for consideration by the entire department.

Departmental Goals

The Reference department outlined several goals they needed to achieve in whatever final plan was developed: (a) a smoothly running reference desk; (b) complete and effective coverage of that desk; (c) oversight of the service provided there; and (d) balance and fairness in the scheduling of individuals, which may seem like secondary needs but which, if perceived as not being met, can cause anger and resentment and adversely effect service.

Other reasons for giving this a try appealed to the department: It provided a measure of flexibility to a staff with many (sometimes conflicting) duties pulling at them. The reference staff also had the beliefs and characteristics of a group of dedicated professionals, working in a climate that fosters both independence and a high degree of cooperation. This proposed procedure appealed to this attitude to a very great degree.

STEPS ALONG THE WAY

With a "third-tier" reference referral system already in place, where questions too specialized for staff at the desk to answer adequately are referred to subject specialists by form, phone, or e-mail, it was considered unnecessary to continue to pair a science specialist with a social science/humanities specialist during a reference shift. Such a complicated addition to everything else that needed to be considered in scheduling a staff this size made the process exceedingly difficult.

Once this was decided, several "trial runs" were made.

Experiment #1: Individual Weekly Self-Scheduling

Sign-up sheets were posted in the department, and individuals scheduled themselves as they were able to get to the sheets. This had significant problems that were immediately apparent, as there was a big rush to get to the sign-up sheets first and this caused some hard feelings among staff unable to get there quickly enough or who couldn't fight their way to the front, who were left with fewer choices and the more unpopular shifts.

This first experiment included an attempt to schedule week by week. Because duties shift in emphasis during a school term, such as heavy faculty liaison at the beginning, instruction happening primarily during the first 2-4 weeks then tapering off, and so on, several people advocated for this. The concept was sound, but in practice most of the staff disliked it. Besides the stress of the rush to get in "first" (with more assertive individuals often obtaining the most desirable schedules), weekly scheduling made it so that the staff would need to go through the process week after week. It was also immediately apparent that doing different schedules for several weeks at the same time was unwieldy and confusing. To try to ease these drawbacks the change was soon made to signing up for a regular term-long schedule.

Experiment #2: Individual Self-Scheduling a Term-Long Schedule

This next step was a variation on the first. A weekly schedule would be established, and this would be followed for all ten weeks of the term. The loss of the weekly flexibility was viewed as justified by the elimination of a great deal of confusion and frustration inherent in so many staff members trying to do ten schedules at once, but it did not relieve the basic problem of those unable to get to the sign-up sheets in time to obtain their choice of shifts, or the "feeding frenzy" (as more than one staff member put it) of people mobbing the table where the sheets were placed. In addition, staff who were not able to get a workable schedule spent a lot of time negotiating later with coworkers to trade shifts.

Experiment #3: Group Scheduling

One member of the Reference Center Management Team then proposed the idea of holding a large scheduling meeting when staff would come together to hammer a schedule out within the group. Negotiation for shifts could take place at one time with everyone together. Sign-up sheets were quickly abandoned under this process in favor of a coordinator filling out a "master schedule" on the whiteboard. Staff took it in turns to claim shifts. The advantages of this were immediately felt: Everyone could see at the same time where the spaces were in the schedule, and the "feeding frenzy" of a large group of people trying to grab a sign-up sheet was eliminated.

Despite some rough spots, this worked well from the beginning. The group discovered that it was quick and relatively painless. At first, things were hectic, as staff who may have begun by conducting themselves in an orderly fashion often got somewhat out of hand as the stress of obtaining the shifts they wanted mounted during the meeting. But over the course of several terms the initial procedure was refined, and currently the department can often schedule everyone for an entire term in 30 minutes.

Development of the Procedure: Setting Ground Rules

For the process to work, agreement had to be reached among staff on the procedures that would be followed. The following concepts were agreed upon by the members of the department:

1. The scheduling meetings would be held during the regular department meeting time. Getting a large staff with many other obliga-

tions together at one time had proved to be extremely difficult. The department meeting was already a protected time for reference staff so the largest number of people would be able to be present then with the least effort.

2. Even though a mix of faculty and classified workers staff the reference desk, it was decided that only the professional library faculty would work evenings and weekends. Not only did this have library tradition behind it, but it also addressed matters of accountability and responsibility–usually the reference librarian is the only faculty in the building during these hours. There was also some difficulty with the contracts of the Reference classified staff, which made evening and weekend duty difficult to schedule and remain within the articles of the contract.

3. In the interests of harmony and employee morale, every effort would be made to give everyone their first shift choice.

DUTY OFFICER

Another task that was accomplished was to arrange someone to be responsible for the smooth running of the services at the reference desk. When budget-driven administrative reorganization eliminated several middle-management positions, the concept of the Duty Officer was borrowed from the military and the Peace Corps as a way for overseeing weekly reference desk service without a desk manager. This was a shared task of all librarians working the reference desk with a different librarian each week taking on a list of responsibilities. (See Appendix A: Role of Duty Officer and Duty Officer Checklist.) This provided for steady management of the desk, with the time and effort each person needed to put into keeping things running minimized. Several other benefits grew from this necessity, as it contributed to staff development by giving reference librarians some management responsibilities and instilling in the members of the reference team a sense of ownership of desk services, inspiring them to care more about how things functioned. "I think it is a great way to ensure every librarian has an opportunity to be involved in the details of caring for the desk," one employee observed. "In fact, I would argue that it is one of the main reasons why . . . [OSU has] such a strong commitment from everyone that taking care of the desk is important."

With the institution of group scheduling, sign-up for "Duty Officer" weeks was eventually folded into the scheduling, and the responsibility for seeing that holes were filled in the desk schedule for their duty week was added to the list of responsibilities of the Duty Officer.

THE FLEXIBILITY TO MAKE IT WORK

Since this was an entirely new way of doing things for the people involved, many changes and adjustments had to take place to arrive at the current system. The procedure continues to be tweaked and adjusted to accommodate changes in the circumstances of the department. (See Appendix B: Reference Desk Scheduling Procedures and Timeline.)

Things go more smoothly if the scheduling group reminds everyone of the procedure before people begin to claim shifts. People bring their personal schedules along to the meeting to aid them in the process, have been informed by the Head of Reference how many hours per week they will need to sign up for, and keep track for themselves as they go through the process. The individuals in charge of the scheduling meeting have to be scrupulously fair in giving everyone a chance at getting their first choice of shift. Once this is done to everyone's satisfaction, the negotiations start for the remaining shifts, with people trading and rearranging until all shifts are filled and everyone has agreed to the schedule.

Very early in the process everyone realized that it was advisable to fill evening hours before scheduling the regular daytime shifts. The evenings are 3-hour shifts rather than the 2-hour shifts standard during the day, and are harder to fill than daytime hours. Interested librarians often didn't have three hours left to allocate if these were left to the end, or had already signed up for early hours that day (creating an undesirable split shift). There is much group negotiation here, and people are aware of the "fairness" issue in sharing the burden (i.e., not making the same librarians work evenings every term–unless of course they prefer to as some do). So far, there have always been enough people willing to take these hours that mandating that all librarians work evenings has not been necessary.

Although evening hours were always done at the scheduling meeting, weekend and Duty Officer shifts, being irregular, were filled using a sign-up sheet. While there has been some back-and-forth about this, currently these shifts are also scheduled at the meeting, as the previous method came to be regarded as an extra step most of the staff considered unnecessary.

At the suggestion of several librarians, another recent change was made. This was to fill Duty Officer weeks before doing weekend scheduling, and then to give the Duty Officer his/her preferred shift on that weekend. Since the Duty Officers must remain "on call" during that weekend it was considered fair to let them have first choice of one or two of these shifts. Since OSU is on a quarterly rather than a semester system, there are generally more librarians than weeks in a term, so not everyone will have a Duty Officer week every term. In this case those people take on one of the extra weekend shifts, which never divide evenly among the number of librarians available.

One major test of the flexibility of the system was the incorporation of scheduling a second service point: the Government Information/Maps (GIM) reference desk. With the major re-visioning of reference services that went hand-in-hand with the complete remodel of existing facilities in 1999, these once-separate departments have been incorporated into a reorganized Reference and Instruction Department. Most technical service responsibility for document and map materials was moved into the Technical Services division, along with several personnel who previously staffed the GIM desk. This shifting made cross-training reference staff to cover hours at the GIM desk imperative. The subject specialists from government documents and maps were trained for and included in the schedule for the main desk, and at the same time several members of the reference staff were trained each term in maps and documents reference and rotated into the GIM desk schedule. After three terms everyone had been cross-trained, and hours for both desks were combined and scheduled at the same scheduling meeting. It works smoothly, as the subject specialists for documents and maps are still available within the 3rd-tier reference referral system to answer the toughest questions.

Another adjustment to the scheduling system was made when a reference specialist/technical writer was hired to work half time at the reference desk. When trying to schedule his 20 hours during a regular scheduling meeting (when others had no more than eight hours) caused some difficulties, it was decided scheduling would be easier for everyone if half of his hours were pre-scheduled, and the rest done at the meeting. In addition to a smoother-running meeting, this guaranteed the technical writer the large blocks of uninterrupted time he needed to do his writing.

One practice which has caused growing tension within the department, and which has been reinforced by the experience of group self-scheduling, is that of covering each other's desk hours. The new term-long schedule, while relieving the stresses of building a new schedule week after week, still left the problem of unanticipated demands cropping up during the term. Because the reference staff is a collegial and cooperative group of people, when other demands took someone away from the desk during scheduled hours there was seldom a problem finding a colleague to volunteer to cover. But with responsibilities of faculty liaison, library instruction duties, conference attendance, and research and publication increasing, this volunteering had been a growing burden on others who could find it adversely impacting their own time needs. It was increasingly evident that " . . . the need to adjust frequently to other staff members' unanticipated absences creates a strain" (Neville, 1982). To help relieve this stress, the department has recently managed to arrange funding to create a pool of "on-call librarians," well-trained general reference specialists who can come in on relatively short notice, which significantly simplified adjusting for major conference times and long- and short-term absences of any sort. This group also covers the desk during the scheduling meeting; before this, one staff member volunteered to cover the desk and her desk hours were pre-scheduled. With the temporary coverage now available this is no longer necessary. While the program is still in its early stages, it has so far been a tremendous success and will be continued for as long as funding can be obtained.

HOW WELL DOES IT ALL WORK?

Several staff members mention that they feel some tension and anxiety at scheduling meetings. Negotiations between employees for shifts can sometimes get a little hot. "There was much negotiation and sometimes I sensed some bad vibes in the air," one librarian stated. There is an advantage, however, in having more than one person involved in the planning. "We had several people involved in the pre-meeting as well which meant that one person could not be held responsible for messing everyone up."

To work well, as many reference staff as possible must be at the scheduling meeting. Putting it on the agenda at the beginning of a regular departmental meeting, which all staff already attend, to some extent assures this. However, there are usually some absences, and those who miss the scheduling meeting can feel disadvantaged and unfairly denied the hours they prefer while others get the most desirable shifts. To deal with this a proxy system was recently formally instituted, where the staff member who will be absent finds another to represent them at the scheduling meeting. That representative takes responsibility for getting the absent person a workable and desirable schedule. If the absence is unforeseen (such as a sudden illness or family emergency), a member of the scheduling group will review the employee's schedule from the previous term and use that as a guide to represent that person at the meeting. In either case, everyone recognizes that some negotiation will need to take place later and perhaps shifts traded.

Several hours of preparation time are still involved in matching total number of hours needing coverage at two desks with how many hours each staff member is responsible for, taking special circumstances (i.e., an unusually heavy teaching commitment that term, a promotion and tenure dossier due, serious illnesses, or other extended absences) into consideration that will force a reduction in some people's hours. There is also some post-scheduling work involved in constructing the final schedule, and copying and distributing it. In some places this can be taken care of by a secretary or other clerical support personnel; during the time the Reference Department had no support staff, the scheduling group did this. One simplification recently instituted is placing a password-protected weekly schedule on the library's intranet, for staff to access from their desk or home computer. This also makes posting changes easier. Input onto the schedule grid has been switched from a whiteboard to an overhead, making it simpler for office support personnel to enter the information onto the master schedule on the computer. Directly entering the data onto a spreadsheet at the scheduling meeting (using a laptop with an overhead projection system) is also being explored but has not yet been instituted.

STAFF OPINIONS

The Valley Library has been working under this procedure for several years, and most staff find it to be the most desirable way of creating a schedule. They believe that the positive aspects of this procedure far outweigh the negatives. The advantages most often mentioned by the staff:

- *Time.* This process is much speedier. Everything (or nearly everything) is settled during the scheduling meeting rather than dragging on over the course of several days or weeks as a scheduling manager tweaks and adjusts the schedule in response to individuals' needs and requests.

- *Responsibility*. Each staff member takes responsibility for himself; things that a scheduler used to be expected to discover and work into the schedule are managed by individuals in this system. This is regarded as the most beneficial aspect of the entire procedure: Reference staff feel that they have a say in their own work lives and input in the quality of service. There is a high degree of responsibility among librarians; the staff care very much about fairness and service.
- *Ownership*. The reference staff member feels ownership of his or her own schedule and is more likely to be satisfied with it. Often when a single person creates a schedule for many, there is resentment toward the scheduler if the staff person draws an unfavorable shift. "No matter how well one can juggle, the schedule may end up making people angry" (Stelk & Lu, 1997). With group scheduling, someone might be unhappy with a shift but accept that this happens to everyone at one time or another, and the resentment is considerably lessened or absent altogether. Everyone is aware that the schedule will only exist for one term at a time, so if someone is "stuck" with a shift or a desk partner that is undesirable to them and unable to make a trade, they know that it *will* change after a few weeks. Some people would like to have the same schedule each term, and others would like to see it change every week, but most like being able to adjust it; they feel it provides a good balance.
- *Preference of hours*. People who prefer late hours and others who like early mornings tend to balance out among the staff, so there are seldom "undesirable" hours left over when staff are allowed to set their own schedules. People seldom are required to work at hours that are unsuitable to them.
- *Weekend flexibility*. People also seem to like that weekend scheduling is considered separate from the daily scheduling; when everyone knows that all librarians will have a roughly equal number of "undesirable" weekend shifts no one feels imposed upon.
- *Ease of negotiation*. It is more convenient to make compromises and negotiations in a large scheduling meeting than having to do it all one-on-one during several days.
- *Enhanced collegiality*. The cooperative nature of the work environment is enhanced, and this carries over into other aspects of departmental work relationships. For example, the department has

become very adept at group scheduling of other kinds of tasks. This became apparent recently when the department took on a much larger role in providing library instruction to the freshman writing (Writing 121) course and decided to apply the desk scheduling procedure to that schedule as well:

> I hope we all appreciate just how well this scheduling has gone. Many thanks to the background work of the Instruction Work Group. But also, many thanks to the department and Reference Services Work Group which has made us really rather skilled at the concept of group scheduling. I mean, if someone asked you how long it would take to get 15 librarians to schedule themselves to teach 28 sections of an entirely new course, would you have guessed 23 minutes (including time for some people to play a game of hangman)? (Bonnie Avery, Acting Head of Reference)

While everyone felt that they had begun this venture with an already well-developed team outlook, their practice at group desk scheduling has nurtured and reinforced it even further. (See Figure 1 for a sample desk schedule at OSU.)

WHAT A LIBRARY NEEDS TO IMPLEMENT IT AND MAKE IT WORK

OSU Libraries has been working for many years in a culture of cooperative team management, and experience and training may have made the change to this kind of unusual scheduling system smoother than it might have been in a more traditional management structure. But even in a traditional hierarchy this could be successfully implemented.

Support from the department head is critical. It requires a certain level of willingness to release some control over the desk schedule to the people who work the schedule. Much also depends upon how much the reference department might desire to gain more control over their schedule.

Since this is a cooperative model, procedures must be clearly stated in a written document and the team must agree to support it. Consensus is an integral requirement.

The key requirement for success is flexibility. The group should feel free to adjust the procedure as needed; ongoing assessment of the process is important and, again, there must be consensus over the changes.

FIGURE 1. Sample Desk Schedule

	Trades		Subs		Need to cover	

April 13-19 Duty Officer Valery King 7-7XXX

	Saturday Apr 13		Sunday Apr 14		Monday Apr 15			Tuesday Apr 16		
	GIM	REF	GIM	REF	GIM	REF	Back up	GIM	REF	Back up
8-9						Paula M.	Cindy S.		Cheryl M.	Carrie O.
9-10					Mary C.	Paula M.	Cindy S.	Cindy S.	Cheryl M.	Carrie O.
10-11	Student	Cheryl M.	Student	Loretta R.	May C.	Garry B.	Anne C.	Joe T.	David J.	Garry B.
11-noon	Student	Cheryl M.	Student	Loretta R.	May C.	Garry B.	Anne C.	Joe T.	David J.	Garry B.
noon-1	Student	Cheryl M.	Student	Loretta R.	May C.	Valery K.	John M.	Valery K.	Laurel M.	Paula M.
1-2	Student	Cheryl M.	Student	Loretta R.	Carrie O	Joe T.	Garry B.	Student	Kristen G.	Russ R.
2-3	Student	Valery K.	Student	David J.	Carrie O	Joe T.	Garry B.	Student	Kristen G.	Russ R.
3-4	Student	Valery K.	Student	David J.	David J.	Mary C.	Bryan M.	John M.	Laurel M.	Joe T.
4-5	Student	Valery K.	Student	David J.	David J.	Mary C.	Bryan M.	John M.	Laurel M.	Joe T.
5-6	Student	Valery K.	Student	David J.	Student	Arlene C.		Student	Loretta R.	
6-7			Student	Joe T.	Student	Arlene C.		Student	Loretta R.	

CHALLENGES FOR THE FUTURE

The current digital revolution taking place in libraries in general is impacting how reference services are delivered. OSU libraries, like many other libraries throughout the world, is feeling the pressure to provide digital delivery of reference services. While still in the earliest planning and decision stages, an electronically delivered reference service is looming on OSU's horizon. The department is confident that the current self-scheduling system will be able to adapt to scheduling a virtual service as well as it did for the additional Government Information and Maps desk and the Writing 121 teaching schedule.

CONCLUSION

The Reference staff is committed to this form of scheduling and believe it is the best way of achieving both fairness in their schedules and the best service at the desk. People in the department–not only the librarians, but Reference's classified staff and support personnel as well–feel that they have some control and responsibility for the smooth running of the reference desks and are more committed to it. While such a system may not work for every institution, it can work well in an environment with committed and dedicated personnel working cooperatively, with the support of the Head of Reference and the library administration. What began as an experiment to relieve a heavy burden from a single employee has turned into a method of empowering reference professionals.

REFERENCES

Butcher, Karyle S. "Total Quality Management: The Oregon State University Library's experience." *Journal of Library Administration*, 18 (1-2) (1993): 45-56.
_____. "Decision Making in a Team Environment." *Library Administration & Management* 11 (Fall 1997): 222-30.
_____ and Kinch, Michael P. "Who Calls the Shots? The Politics of Reference Reorganization." *The Journal of Academic Librarianship*, 16 (5) (1990): 280-84.
Cornick, Donna and Owen, Willy. "Microcomputer Scheduling of Reference Desk Staff." *RQ* 28 (Fall 1988): 46-53.
Davidson, Jeanne and Rusk, Cherie. "Creating a University Web in a Team Environment." *Journal of Academic Librarianship* (July 1996): 302-05.
Dennison, Russel F. "Usage-Based Staffing of the Reference Desk: A Statistical Approach." *Reference & User Services Quarterly* 39 (2) (1999): 158-65.
King, Geraldine B. "The Management of Reference Services." *RQ* 26 (Summer 1987): 407-9.
Neville, Sandra H. "Day to Day Management of Reference Services." *The Reference Librarian* 3 (Spring 1982): 15-27.
Stelk, Roger and Lu, Suping. "Eight Days a Week: The Art of Reference Desk Scheduling." Co-published simultaneously in *The Reference Librarian* 59 (1997): 37-50; and in *Philosophies of Reference Service* edited by Celia Hales Mabry. The Haworth Press, Inc., 1988. 37-50.

APPENDIX A

ROLE OF DUTY OFFICER

Assumptions

The role of Duty Officer is based on the model of weekly rotation of management responsibilities for the Reference Division. During the week a person serves as Duty Officer he/she acts not as an individual librarian, but as the person with the ultimate responsibility for keeping the Reference Desk functioning smoothly and as the person who agrees to make short term public service decisions.

The role of Duty Officer will be shared equally by all tenured and tenure-track librarians in the Reference Division, with the exception of the Distance Education Librarian, and will be in addition to his/her regular duties that week.

Specific Duties of Duty Officer

1. Check weekly reference desk schedule a few days in advance. Remind weekend staff of the hours they agreed to work. Consult with Reference Support to fill daytime desk vacancies from the on-call librarian pool. Send out report of desk coverage vacancies for evening/weekend shifts and daytime shifts that cannot be filled from the on-call pool and solicit persons to fill them. It is the Duty Officer's responsibility to see that the reference desk is staffed all the hours scheduled.

2. In case of illness or other unanticipated absences, contact Reference Support to see if it is possible to have an on-call staff member cover the hours. If not, solicit volunteers. If substitutes cannot be found, the Duty Officer will be responsible for personally staffing the desk.

3. Check the department calendar and post the department's absences for the day on the whiteboard at the Reference Desk each morning.

4. Serve as point person for other Library departments who need to communicate with Reference staff regarding public service staffing changes, emergencies, etc. (for example, staff absences in Circulation affecting evening or weekend coverage). Take responsibility for communicating this information to those who need to know.

5. Arrange for signs to be put up in advance when there is PLANNED downtime for OASIS, ORBIS or the Library or University Computing Networks. Notification of planned downtime is usually received a few days in advance. Signs should be prepared and mounted by Reference support staff,

coordinated by Duty Officer, and removed when no longer needed. Posting and removal of signs for unanticipated downtime will be done by Reference or Technical Assistance Desk staff on an as-needed basis.

6. Serve as point person and arrange for posting and removal of signs for such things as emergency library closures or temporary or unscheduled closures of reference desk by personally posting signs or delegating to office support staff.

Duties of Reference Support in Regard to Duty Officer

1. Prepare list of Duty Officers for the term or intersession. All tenured or tenure-track librarians will sign up for Duty Officer as part of Reference Desk duty.
2. At the beginning of each term, send list of Duty Officers to Access Services, Library Administration, and Library Automation, and post list in Reference office.
3. Arrange for desk coverage by on-call librarians as needed when requested by Duty Officer (usually in cases of unexpected absences).

Expectations of Duty Officers

1. The weekly Duty Officer "shift" runs from Saturday through Friday.
2. In the spirit of shared management, during the week prior to and the week you are Duty Officer, take responsibility for reading e-mail and other notices in terms of how the running of Information Commons/Reference/Public Services might be affected on a daily basis. Take responsibility to respond appropriately not as an individual, but as the person "in charge" of Reference for that time period.
3. In order to be able to respond to emergencies affecting reference desk coverage, expect that you may be contacted at home by phone if the situation warrants immediate action, e.g., a weekend Reference Desk staffer does not show up for his/her shift.
4. Responsibilities as Duty Officer will be in addition to regularly scheduled Reference Desk duty that week.

Expectations of Reference Desk Staff

Classified, unclassified and on-call staff who cannot work during their scheduled desk hours should do the following:

1. Anticipated Absences (conferences, vacations, medical appointments, etc.). Contact Reference Support and the Duty Officer for the week(s) of

your absences with a list of desk times you cannot cover, as far in advance as is possible. Reference Support will arrange for on-call staff members to cover your hours. If on-call staff members are not available, the Duty Officer will solicit volunteers to cover the hours.

2. Unanticipated Absences (sudden illness, family emergency, etc.). Notify the Duty Officer that you will not be able to work a specific shift or shifts. The Duty Officer will contact Reference Support to see if it is possible to have an on-call staff member cover your hours. If not, the Duty Officer will solicit volunteers. If you cannot contact the Duty Officer directly, call the reference phone number. *General Rule*: In e-mail communications concerning any issue mentioned above, copy both Reference Support and the Duty Officer as a matter of course.

See also: Duty Officer Checklist (document revised 7/20/2001, vk)

Duty Officer Checklist

Duty Officer shift begins on Friday afternoon and ends at 5 pm the following Friday.

NOTE ON ARRANGING ON-CALL LIBRARIAN COVERAGE: When an absence occurs, ask Reference Support to find on-call staff to fill the vacancy. If none are available, solicit volunteers as before.

On-call staff, classified staff and non-tenure-track faculty do not fill in evening or weekend shifts; you must find a librarian to do these.

Week in Advance

Check weekly reference desk schedule for your shift. Note any vacancies and obtain on-call coverage if possible; if unavailable, solicit regular reference staff to fill them.

Week of Your Shift

- Late Friday afternoon: photocopy and post next week's schedule at all public service desks–Reference, Circulation, and GIM–and the reference office bulletin board.
- Friday: check with persons scheduled to work weekend shifts to be sure they remember they are working the weekend.

- Each afternoon: post absences for next day on the message whiteboard at the reference desk. (This can be done the next morning if you are in early.) 8:00 am reference person will add any call-in absences.
- Early each morning: check your e-mail and phone messages for emergency absences. Arrange on-call librarian coverage or solicit regular staff to fill these and other absences which arise during week of your shift.

As Needed During Your Shift

- Serve as point person for other Library depts. who need to communicate with Reference staff regarding public service changes, emergencies, etc.
- Arrange for signs to be prepared and put up in advance when there is PLANNED downtime for OASIS, ORBIS, or the library or University Computing Networks.
- Serve as point person for posting and removal of signs for such things as emergency library closures or temporary closures of reference desk.

This information does not replace the full Duty Officer document, but is meant as a quick checklist of the major duties.

(This page revised 7/20/2001, vk)

APPENDIX B

REFERENCE DESK SCHEDULING PROCEDURES AND TIMELINE

Scheduling for Fall, Winter or Spring Term

1. By the end of the 9th week of the prior term, people who want to have reduced desk hours or opt out of desk duty completely for the upcoming term need to have received approval from Head of Reference. Reference Services Workgroup designated scheduling manager will send e-mail reminding staff of this deadline during the 8th week.
2. During the 10th week (dead week), scheduling manager contacts Head of Reference to ascertain who is eligible for weekly desk hours (and for how many), weekend desk hours and Duty Officer list for the upcoming term.

3. Also during the 10th week scheduling manager calculates the number of hours to be covered per week on Reference and GIM desks. (NOTE: The hours of 8-5 Monday through Friday include a back-up librarian position at the Reference desk; the GIM desk does not. There are no back-up positions in the evenings.) This information is used to calculate the full-time and half-time obligations. Weekends to be covered are divided into 4 hour shifts and total shifts are divided equally among eligible weekend librarians. If this division cannot be made equally, any librarian not signing up for a Duty Officer spot may be asked to do an extra weekend shift. Scheduling manager sends this information out via e-mail so people can prepare to sign up.

4. A group scheduling meeting is held during the 11th week (finals) for people to choose desk hours. Both Reference Desk and GIM Desk hours are scheduled at this time. Any staff member who cannot attend the meeting should arrange for a representative to sign up for them and provide that representative with information about their preferred desk hours and hours they are unable to work at the desk. [Garry who has a greater number of desk hours to fill than the rest of the staff signs up previous to the scheduling meeting and covers the Reference desk during the meeting. If he is unable to cover the desk, the person who does is allowed to sign up in advance.]

5. Duty Officer and weekend shifts are also scheduled at this time. Only librarians fill weekend and Duty Officer positions (no classified or non-ranked faculty). Duty Officer has first choice of shifts for that weekend. Weekend shifts start the Saturday before the first day of classes; the Reference desk is not staffed the weekend following Finals week (for desk scheduling purposes this is considered part of Intersession).

6. After the scheduling meeting a draft of the weekly schedule is posted. People have one week to trade or adjust their selections. After this, regular weekly printouts for the entire term are made, with weekend and Duty Officers listed. Files for past and current terms are saved in the S:\reference\schedule directory in WordPerfect format.

Scheduling for Summer Term and Intersessions

1. By the end of the 9th week of the prior term, intersession hours to be covered are calculated. GIM desk during intersession is covered by student workers; Reference desk is not staffed on weekends during intersession, nor is there is a back-up librarian assigned during that week. Summer and intersession hours are divided equally among eligible staff–no full-time or half-time categories.

2. Head of Reference informs the scheduling manager how many people are eligible for desk coverage.

3. At beginning of 10th week scheduling manager informs staff how many hours each person needs to sign up for during the entire intersession. Sheets are posted and staff sign up throughout 10th week. There is no group scheduling meeting. Intersession schedules are posted by the middle of the 11th week.

4. For Summer schedule, scheduling manager informs staff how many hours each person needs to sign up for during the summer weekdays and weekday evenings. Weekend hours are divided into shifts and all staff sign up for an equal number of weekend shifts. There is no group scheduling meeting.

5. For Summer or intersession, Duty Officers sign up on the scheduling sheets.

[amended 3/21/01–vk]

Cooperation in a Multi-Faceted Reference Department: Blending Resources, Personnel, and Services of Reference, Instruction, Interlibrary Loan, and Government Documents

Della H. Darby
Lori A. Northrup
Carla T. Waddell
Heather F. Watters

SUMMARY. Cooperative reference is a valuable approach to serving patrons as well as a means of expanding one's professional knowledge. Members of the reference unit actively participate in cooperative reference for answering patrons' tougher queries, bibliographic instruction, and reference collection development. The cooperative efforts of our

---

Della H. Darby (E-mail: dhdarby@samford.edu) is Reference Librarian; Lori A. Northrup (E-mail: lanorthr@samford.edu) is Reference Librarian; Carla T. Waddell (E-mail: ctwaddel@samford.edu) is Reference and Instruction Librarian, all at Samford University Library, 800 Lakeshore Parkway, Birmingham, AL 35229. Heather F. Watters can be reached at 1308 Shelby County Highway 1, Bessemer, AL 35022 (E-mail: heatherann@wwisp.com). At the time this was written, she was Reference and Government Documents Librarian, Samford University Library, Birmingham, AL.

[Haworth co-indexing entry note]: "Cooperation in a Multi-Faceted Reference Department: Blending Resources, Personnel, and Services of Reference, Instruction, Interlibrary Loan, and Government Documents." Darby et al. Co-published simultaneously in *The Reference Librarian* (The Haworth Information Press, an imprint of The Haworth Press, Inc.) No. 83/84, 2003, pp. 119-130; and: *Cooperative Reference: Social Interaction in the Workplace* (ed: Celia Hales Mabry) The Haworth Information Press, an imprint of The Haworth Press, Inc., 2003, pp. 119-130. Single or multiple copies of this article are available for a fee from The Haworth Document Delivery Service [1-800-HAWORTH, 9:00 a.m. - 5:00 p.m. (EST). E-mail address: docdelivery@haworthpress.com].

Digital Object Identifier: 10.1300J120v40n83_10

unit have expanded our ability to find better information faster. Cooperative reference extends to all librarians within the University Library as
each librarian serves in a rotation to staff the reference desk on nights and
weekends. Some of the benefits of practicing cooperative reference are
the following: providing a balanced and sometimes more complete answer to a reference question; increasing the knowledge of the reference
staff by sharing experiences; and increasing morale and support for the
reference staff. All of this is accomplished by doing what librarians do
best: sharing. Successful cooperative reference relies upon good communication within the department, respect for colleagues, flexibility, and
commitment to serving our patrons. *[Article copies available for a fee from
The Haworth Document Delivery Service: 1-800-HAWORTH. E-mail address:
<docdelivery@haworthpress.com> Website: <http://www.HaworthPress.com> © 2003
by The Haworth Press, Inc. All rights reserved.]*

KEYWORDS. Cooperation, collaboration, reference, interlibrary loan,
government documents

INTRODUCTION

Samford University is a small- to medium-sized institution, with
about 2,900 undergraduate and 1,500 graduate students. The campus has
four information units: the University Library, the Law Library, the Education Curriculum Center, and the Drug Information Center. The University Library is the primary information center for all disciplines
except Law. Within the Reference Department, which is one of several
University Library departments, four full-time librarians, two full-time
paraprofessionals, and several student assistants are responsible for
general reference, government documents reference, and interlibrary
loan functions. Samford's reference staff is in a unique position in that
five of these staff members have been at the University for two years or
less. In such a new environment, members have tended in the past to
congregate and discuss departmental business; this habit of conspiracy
bled naturally into the reference transactions and other resultant functions of the department. As an increasingly larger and ever newer staff
negotiated the management of the various reference functions, they created a nurturing cooperative reference environment.

Cooperative reference is a valuable approach to serving patrons as
well as a means of expanding one's own professional knowledge. Mem-

bers of the unit actively participate in cooperative reference not only for answering patrons' tougher queries but for bibliographic instruction, materials evaluation, and reference collection development as well. The cooperative efforts in our unit have expanded our ability to find better information faster. The physical structure of the unit lends itself to collaboration with colleagues. Cooperative reference is not only practiced within our unit; it extends to all librarians within the University Library. Each librarian serves in a rotation to cover the reference desk on nights and weekends. Despite being asked to give time to another department, the librarians have a cooperative and flexible attitude. Several have remarked upon the benefit of having contact with our patrons. Some of the benefits of practicing cooperative reference are the following: providing a balanced answer to a reference question (and sometimes a more complete answer); increasing the knowledge of the reference staff by sharing experiences; and increasing morale and support for the reference staff. All of this is accomplished by doing what librarians do best: sharing. Successful cooperative reference relies upon good communication within the department, respect for colleagues, flexibility, and commitment to serving our patrons.

THE LAYOUT

Samford University Library's Reference Department, Government Documents Department, and Interlibrary Loan Department occupy one floor in the University Library building. The Interlibrary Loan Department and the Reference Department are next to each other with the Government Documents Department across from them. Stacks and open floor space separate each of these areas, but distances are not great, and members often congregate in the middle of the Reference desk area, which is equidistant from the other two departments. Since reference staff have small offices, and there are only a few chairs in the desk area, members often stand and talk, or move chairs from the offices into a circle to discuss recent meetings or developments, or to negotiate the best paths to answers for reference questions that have been presented. This arrangement lends itself nicely to both impromptu and planned meetings. The area around the reference desk and offices is generally open, so that staff members can see each other passing by or moving about and can quickly engage each other. Another recent innovation has been the adoption of chat technology among the reference staff. Rather than inhibit socializing, as might be feared, chatting makes it easier to call meetings in the reference area. Because we are distributed around a large physical area, it also allows us to know when someone is in her office. Members do not find it useful for lengthy discussions, but as a catalyst to them.

REFERENCE

Samford has not yet instituted virtual reference, though we hope to do so this fall. As it stands now, reference interviews take place in person and by telephone, and some reference queries are handled by e-mail via our Ask-a-Librarian service. In all three instances, but primarily in telephone and e-mail reference, cooperative reference plays a significant role.

The reference desk, during normal fall and spring semester hours, is staffed from 8:00 a.m. to 9:00 p.m. by librarians, who work in shifts of two to three hours. During the day shifts (i.e., from 8:00 a.m. to 4:30 p.m.), librarians at the desk are never far from other staff members, who may be in their offices or in the open department area. As Olszak aptly noted, close proximity enables overhearing conversations between colleagues. Staff who are nearby can often infer that a colleague may be floundering, or that a patron is dissatisfied (1991). Should the staff member on duty not ask for help, colleagues may step in anyway, with advice or with a previously used resource. When the staff member lacks particular expertise or the confidence to proceed with the question, she may confer immediately with her colleagues. Very often, other staff members can lend their knowledge of the subject area, or can recount ways in which the question has been handled in the past. This method of casting about for answers before heading into the stacks or out into cyberspace very often results in a much more efficient response. When longer discussion is needed, librarians often take the name and number or e-mail address of the student and deliver an answer or a resource at a later time. This too allows for discussion and demonstration among all staff who are present. Such situational and informal coaching by colleagues, while it could be viewed as threatening or interfering behavior (Huling, 1999), is welcomed by the reference staff, as it leads to more confident interviewing behaviors in the future, and, ultimately, to better patron service. Even when librarians feel that they have adequately handled a reference interview, discussion of the question(s) often takes place afterward, in the spirit of sharing knowledge for better service.

In an ideal setting, there would always be colleagues with whom to confer, and patrons who were supremely patient; as in most academic situations, however, staffing the reference desk often means working alone, and working with several patrons at once. When conversation is not possible, staff can rely on written communication to keep them informed and ready for possibly daunting questions. At the reference desk, a log is maintained that contains questions and possible answers and strategies for difficult or frequent questions (what we call "repeaters"). When possible, we also attach copies of current assignments with notes regarding successful search strategies. The purpose of the log is to provide assistance to those who were not present when the questions were presented. It has proven to be especially helpful to the librarians from other units who staff the desk during nights and weekends.

Telephone reference and e-mail reference are perfect opportunities for cooperative reference work. Unlike face-to-face interviews, more time is allowed and accepted for the response. These questions often require clarification of the policies of other departments, so they provide another opportunity to draw others into the fray. The varied experiences of staff members in other departments, especially those of senior staff members, can help reference staff further define their own departmental practices in light of established organizational policies and past practices in other departments (Nofsinger and Lee, 1994). The implicitly longer nature of telephone and e-mail transactions means that librarians have more time for interaction and communication. These types of questions benefit not only the patron, who is likely to get a more thorough response, but also the department as a whole.

In addition to staffing the reference desk, all reference librarians participate in the creation and maintenance of web pages that serve as instruction and pathfinder surrogates for our patrons. We jointly developed a template for subject-specific pages that includes electronic databases, reference materials, and Internet resources. These pages often serve as the outline for subject-specific instruction sessions. They also provide guidance for the non-reference librarians and students who staff the reference desk during nights and weekends. The instruction librarian, in consultation with other members of the reference unit, developed "How Do I?" guides to further aid patrons in negotiating the complexities of research. The government documents librarian maintains a set of pages that simplifies both patrons' and librarians' searches for answers in the vast amount of information produced by the federal government. Two members of the reference unit serve on the library web team and seek input from other members of the unit regarding changes both before and after they are implemented.

GOVERNMENT DOCUMENTS

The success of the Government Documents Department relies upon cooperative reference. The documents collection is accessible to the public at all hours of library operation. Only two full-time employees staff the collection, making it necessary for the reference librarians in the night and weekend reference desk rotation to be able to answer general document questions. Considering that documents have their own classification scheme and Congressional publications are often challenging to decode, it can sometimes be a puzzling collection, but all librarians on staff have been willing to field document questions. In fact, librarians follow up with the documents librarian when they are unsure if they helped a patron to find the best information, demonstrating a commitment to good reference service. Rather than taking the attitude that government documents "is not their area," the librarians have adopted an attitude of willingness to learn about the collection. Because of this attitude, patrons of Government Documents are served even when the government documents librarian is not available.

Not unlike other academic institutions with a government depository, Samford University's government documents librarian divides her time between the documents collection and the reference desk. This allows the full-time reference librarians time to fulfill other responsibilities beyond answering patron queries while the documents librarian benefits by being exposed to the needs of the patrons and developing her own reference skills. When reference librarians are posed a question related to finding government information, they first help the patron find the information by searching the library's catalog and government web sites. This provides quality service instead of slowing the process by automatically referring the patron to the Government Documents staff. Likewise, when a patron approaches the Government Documents desk with a general reference question, the documents staff answers the question in order to efficiently serve the patron. For more complex questions, the reference librarians consult the documents librarian and see that the patron knows where the documents collection is, often by personal escort. As a result of this team approach, a reference librarian and the documents librarian often work on the same question together. By pooling their resources and experience, the most possible avenues for the information have been explored and questions are answered with confidence.

INSTRUCTION

Cooperation with fellow reference librarians is essential with a one-person instruction team. The cooperation includes sharing the course load; brainstorming for new ideas; proofreading of material; and feedback from each session.

The instruction course load is shared among the reference librarians. The instruction librarian teaches approximately half of the freshman orientation sessions, with the other half being divided among the other reference librarians each semester. The instruction librarian teaches most of the subject-specific sessions unless another librarian has expertise in the area. She creates PowerPoint shows for the freshman sessions so we can basically point and click through an outline for the session. The instruction librarian makes any necessary material such as handouts, worksheets, and PowerPoint shows available in advance so that the other reference librarians can review and edit. We also test new materials on our student assistants to verify their clarity and usability. Feedback from each librarian regarding the sessions they taught is given to the instruction librarian for future use or to make changes within the current plan.

Just this past year, the reference unit worked together to redesign one of the freshman-level core courses. Life-long learning skills (ACRL, 2002), or at least semester-long skills, were inserted into the session. We also included a variety of activities to include the various types of learning skills. The benefits of including the reference librarians in the planning process included the following: (1) increased comfort level regarding the teaching of familiar material; (2) ownership; (3) a greater variety of ideas to choose from; and (4) the shared praise for a successful revision.

Through instruction, the reference librarians at Samford also provide community service and outreach. We teach four to five sessions each summer to a local rehabilitation group. Each group is always a surprise in that the skill levels vary from your average high school hacker to the adult returning student who believes the mouse should be in a trap. Team teaching is, therefore, vital since there are always one or two students that require one-on-one assistance throughout the session. Even with the challenge and chaos, we leave these sessions knowing that a difference was made with at least one student. The ability of all reference librarians to pitch in as needed is essential to a smoothly operating department. Requests for instruction during the summer often occur with short notice and invariably for the time when the instruction librarian is on vacation.

Team teaching is not limited to the rehabilitation group, but is used also for larger classes in the regular schedule of instruction. The larger courses require team teaching due to the number of students. We believe in using hands-on activities, which always create questions. The second librarian assists with the questions and any technical difficulties. With only 50 minutes per session, time is important, and we prefer that the students complete the activity rather than waiting for a question to be answered.

COLLECTION DEVELOPMENT

Collection development is a component for all reference librarian positions at Samford. Because they interact daily with patrons, reference librarians are familiar with patron requests for materials. They are also painfully aware when the collection fails to meet patrons' needs (Intner, 1988). All members of the Reference Department contribute to the collection's direction by recommending new purchases, noting new editions or revisions of materials already in the collection, and suggesting discards. Rather than participating separately in making recommendations to the Collection Development department, each member of the Reference Unit meets and discusses with her peers her suggestions for the collection. This interaction often occurs in the form of casual conversation near the reference desk, and, while a scheduled meeting to discuss these suggestions has recently been instituted, it was the result of conversation that was already taking place. These scheduled meetings most often concern additions to the collection, while more casual encounters seem to accompany discussion of withdrawals.

Reference librarians submit to the Collection Development department materials they would like to see removed from the collection. These suggestions are often the result of reference searches. In the process of answering reference questions, for instance, librarians may note that an updated edition of a work or a newer source of information is needed. Candidates for replacement or withdrawal are brought to the reference desk area where consultation among librarians can take place. The suggesting librarian gives reasons for weeding and/or replacement, and gets feedback from all staff members who are present. Materials are then either returned to the shelf or sent to Collection Development.

Similarly, librarians' suggestions for new titles are discussed in planned monthly meetings of the reference staff. At these meetings, librarians discuss potential additions that they have collected in the period between meetings. A common collection box in the office of the Head of Reference holds suggestion slips between discussions. Following the introduction of a new title, librarians discuss the library's current collection practices in the related areas, past patterns of use, and any relevant faculty or student requests related to a particular item. Such discussions are generally informal and often anecdotal in nature. While these meetings are generally helpful to all the staff, they can be particularly helpful to librarians new to librarianship or to the library and its patrons. Often, in the process of "making a case" for a particular book or database, librarians will talk about past practices in the Department, particular student assignments, or strengths and weaknesses of a similar source.

Together with casual meetings to discuss discards, these meetings encourage collection development and active thought about the collection's direction. They also stimulate spontaneous discussion of recent reference activity, creating for all present a communal knowledge base to be consulted in the future. Because such social interaction is encouraged, librarians are better able to conduct reference interviews, supply guidance to patrons online and in the classroom, and analyze reference resources with regard to the collection.

When new reference materials arrive, they are held in the reference desk area to provide an opportunity for all librarians to evaluate them before they are shelved. This often results in a discussion of the merits and usability of the materials.

PROFESSIONAL DEVELOPMENT

Because of our commitment to continuing quality improvement in resources and services, we recognize the need for continuous growth and development of our skills and professional knowledge. While it is not often possible for all of us to attend every training opportunity, we attempt to allow the majority to participate in the most relevant. We also try to have at least one representative attend less critical functions. Information gained is then shared with other librarians, often in the form of a presentation. The reference coordinator believes strongly in mentoring and growing members of the unit, so she seeks opportunities and financial support for attendance of members at professional conferences and workshops.

MANAGEMENT

The diverse composition of the reference unit provides support for each of the areas that are included. Librarians and support staff are cross-trained and can provide assistance and backup as needed. For instance, reference librarians provide citation verification assistance to the interlibrary loan assistant. During times when student assistants are absent, they assist with catalog checking and deliveries. Librarians provide instruction to the interlibrary loan and government documents assistants in the use of new databases and resources that will enable them to better perform their jobs. The government documents and interlibrary loan assistants provide reference desk coverage when the librarians are committed elsewhere for short periods. The government documents assistant and the reference coordinator serve as back-up to the interlibrary loan assistant. This allows the interlibrary loan assistant to take much needed vacations without interrupting the flow of materials into and out of the library.

Scheduling is greatly simplified because all reference librarians serve equal time at the reference desk and are very flexible about swapping shifts. At the beginning of each semester, the reference coordinator develops a schedule framework and seeks input from the other librarians about its workability. With staff losses and additions and adjustments to the times of desk coverage, the schedule is evaluated and revised to accommodate the preferences of the staff while maintaining the highest level of service for our patrons. During the height of the instruction season, the instruction librarian's hours at the reference desk are reduced and the other librarians share the offset. When one librarian is away for a workshop or conference, the others make up the difference. When all of the reference unit need to be away for an extended period, such as for a professional conference or workshop, librarians from technical services are kind enough to provide desk coverage.

Student assistants are shared throughout the unit. They are trained in at least two areas, so they can be relocated as the workload shifts from one area to another. In government documents, students process and shelve materials and assist with database maintenance. In interlibrary loan, they gather, check out, and package books; scan, fax, and copy articles; and deliver materials to offices on campus. In reference, students shelve reference materials; copy, deliver, and retrieve materials; and staff the reference desk from 9:00 p.m. to midnight. By sharing the student workforce, we not only increase the number of potential work hours for the students, which makes it easier to work around their class schedules, but we improve the knowledge and abilities of our workforce, which makes them more valuable to the library and assists them with their education.

The areas that make up the reference unit are compatible and complementary. The members of the unit represent diverse backgrounds in libraries and other work environments, which have proven to be a great strength. Because reference unit staff share reference duties for all the areas included, patrons are able to receive assistance from anyone they encounter.

Reference librarians assist patrons with placing interlibrary loan requests, which improves the information the interlibrary loan assistant receives. The interlibrary loan assistant (our single "old-timer" and former student) is intimately familiar with the periodical and circulating collections, thus providing all other members of the unit and patrons with a quick answer to where materials are located. The reference coordinator was formerly a technical services librarian and provides elucidation of cataloging and acquisitions practices as needed, as well as the policies and collections of the universities where she was employed. The instruction librarian previously managed a circulation department and provides insight into those activities as well as the policies and collection of a local university library. The reference librarian was employed by the local public library and her insights regarding their collection and policies are often helpful when referring patrons to the public library. The government documents librarian, as expected, is intimately familiar with that collection, so provides in-depth assistance with the documents collection as needed. Her prior and current experience with cataloging are often helpful in interpreting catalog records. She previously directed the library for the Women's Missionary Union and brings her extended knowledge and expertise of religious materials to the fold. The government documents assistant previously owned and managed a bookstore so provides insight into the commercial information seeking behavior of our community.

CONCLUSION

In face-to-face, telephone, e-mail, and electronic reference practice, the Reference Department revolves around open communication. Communication within the unit and with other units in the library is constant and ongoing. Experienced colleagues benefit from new ideas and perspectives that are presented by newly hired, or less experienced staff members; newly hired staff members are able to contribute to and take knowledge from a shared pool of expertise (Nofsinger and Lee, 1994). All members gain knowledge and confidence through shared interactions with library patrons.

At the foundation of this practice of open and nurturing communication is an outstanding service philosophy, which is one of the primary qualities we seek when hiring new employees. Employees are also extremely flexible regarding the assignment of duties and scheduling of activities. Every member of the unit respects the talents and abilities of the other members and their actual and potential contributions to our mission, which is to serve the information needs of our patrons. We value our differences and try to capitalize on them. These traits are essential to the smooth operation of the unit and to the library as a whole as we face ever-increasing changes not only in the multiplicity of formats available, but in the usage patterns and behaviors of our patrons.

REFERENCES

Association of College and Research Libraries, *Information Literacy Competency Standards for Higher Education*, Online. 2002 [Available: http://www.ala.org/acrl/il/toolkit/standards.html] 27 September 2002.

Huling, Nancy (1999), "Peer Reflection: Collegial Coaching and Reference Effectiveness," *The Reference Librarian* no. 66, 61-74.

Intner, Sheila S. (1988), "Collection Development: Necessarily a Shared Enterprise, " *North Carolina Libraries* 46 (Winter), 214-218.

Nofsinger, Mary M. and Lee, Angela S. W. (1994), "Beyond Orientation: The Roles of Senior Librarians in Training Entry-Level Reference Colleagues, " *College and Research Libraries* (March), 161-170.

Why Social Interaction and Good Communication in Academic Libraries Matters

Maria Anna Jankowska
Linnea Marshall

SUMMARY. In these times of extraordinary development in information and communication technologies (ICT) many new tools and services, and traditional tools, such as the catalog, could be developed or enhanced by librarians to effectively support the academic community in teaching and learning. This paper will discuss how social interaction between technical and public service librarians could enhance library services to the academic faculty and students during these demanding times of technologies and information overload. The paper will also point out that the team approach to library services can improve social interaction between librarians when the perpetuation of the traditional academic organizational model is not efficient enough for the faculty and students' need-driven use of information. Rapid changes resulting from ICT demand constant social interaction that would be facilitated by establishing working teams for specific tasks. *[Article copies available for a fee from The Haworth Document Delivery Service: 1-800-HAWORTH. E-mail address: <docdelivery@haworthpress.com> Website: <http://www.HaworthPress.com> © 2003 by The Haworth Press, Inc. All rights reserved.]*

Maria Anna Jankowska (E-mail: majanko@uidaho.edu) is Professor/Reference Librarian, and Linnea Marshall (E-mail: linneam@uidaho.edu) is Assistant Professor/Catalog Librarian, both at University of Idaho Library, P.O. Box 442350, Moscow, ID 83844-2350.

[Haworth co-indexing entry note]: "Why Social Interaction and Good Communication in Academic Libraries Matters." Jankowska, Maria Anna, and Linnea Marshall. Co-published simultaneously in *The Reference Librarian* (The Haworth Information Press, an imprint of The Haworth Press, Inc.) No. 83/84, 2003, pp. 131-144; and: *Cooperative Reference: Social Interaction in the Workplace* (ed: Celia Hales Mabry) The Haworth Information Press, an imprint of The Haworth Press, Inc., 2003, pp. 131-144. Single or multiple copies of this article are available for a fee from The Haworth Document Delivery Service [1-800-HAWORTH, 9:00 a.m. - 5:00 p.m. (EST). E-mail address: docdelivery@haworthpress.com].

KEYWORDS. Social interaction, cooperation, collaboration, team work, public services, technical services, reference librarians, catalog librarians

TECHNOLOGY DEMANDS SOCIAL INTERACTION

Information and communication technologies (ICT) include diverse tools and resources used to communicate, create, disseminate, store, and manage information (Blurton, 1999). All those processes are essential to teaching, research, learning, and the administrative activities of higher education and academic libraries. The global information structure that combines computers, communication networks, and digital systems supplies mechanisms to satisfy the widespread demand for data, information, and knowledge (Jankowska, 2003). A wide access to the information infrastructure has influenced new patterns of searching for information and new information needs among academic faculty and students. A recent study of the information-gathering habits of students and faculty members has found that they first turn to online materials, although most view print as a more reliable source of information (Carlson, 2002). The World Wide Web (Web) has decentralized the information environment and created a non-linear (hypertext) information structure. This structure allows faculty and students to retrieve information at many different levels but also increases the difficulty in finding pertinent information. The Web does not have a controlled vocabulary such as libraries have developed for subject headings. In this time of information overload, faculty and students need efficient and comprehensive access for their information-seeking processes; that requires the cooperative work of both public and technical services librarians.

This cooperative work depends on good communication and social interaction between librarians. The traditional library organizational model, with major divisions for public and technical services, does not provide a common set of values that would be the foundation for effective communication and social interaction. As Robin Mansell (1996) pointed out, "analysis of the determinants of technological changes cannot be divorced from the analysis of institutional changes." In the same way, new information and communication technology cannot be "divorced" from human behaviors and interaction between people.

SOCIAL INTERACTION DEFINED

Consider universities and libraries from an organizational culture approach. An organization is a social construct that is characterized by a set of beliefs and assumptions that define its culture and are shared by the members of the organization. Lacking an articulated mission from the administration, beliefs may be promulgated among the members through their own personal communications among themselves (Budd, 1998). The quantity, quality, and inclusiveness of these personal communications contribute to, or detract from, a unified organizational vision. Lack of communication between the members of any organization could lead to a splintering of purpose and individual actions into unrelated directions and a dissipation of energies and resources with a resultant degeneration in service and product. For public services librarians and technical services librarians to effectively support each other's efforts, they need to embrace a common set of values and goals. Social interaction fosters the development of common values and goals, and aids in the achievement of those goals.

Social interaction was defined by R. J. Rummel (1976) as "the acts, actions, or practices of two or more people mutually oriented towards each other's selves, that is, any behavior that tries to affect or take account of each other's subjective experiences or intentions." Rummel stated that people do not necessarily need to be within sight of each other for social interaction to occur. What is important is that there is a mutual orientation towards each other. Thus Rummel considered friends corresponding with each other to be an example of a social interaction. But in order to be mutual, social interaction must be direct, interactive, and reciprocal.

It is possible to define different levels, or degrees, of social interaction. Social interaction includes actions as simple as small talk to the progressively more complex actions of collegiality, cooperation, and collaboration. Social interaction at each of these levels is important, but the more complex actions have greater impact within an organization. Small talk, though casual and seemingly superficial, serves to create a relaxed environment. It sets a tone of courtesy and a feeling of inclusiveness and community, gives practice to listening, acknowledges an individual's existence, and establishes the basis for ongoing conversation between individuals. Small talk affects the general attitudes within the group. Collegiality similarly affects attitudes but brings forward the process of social interaction to a higher level. Collegiality takes courtesy to respect, community to trust, acknowledgement of an individual's presence to acknowledgement of that individual's contributions, and conversation to consultation and sharing of knowledge. Both small talk and collegiality, by affecting attitudes and the tone of the work place, make possible the higher levels of social interaction, that is, interaction that leads to action. Cooperation and collaboration both require a more active response and result in greater benefits to an organization.

Cooperation occurs when individuals realize the interrelatedness of their decisions and actions–developing an awareness of an organizational ecology of interlinking subsystems–and purposefully act to coordinate their efforts to help alleviate difficulties or facilitate processes within another subsystem. This requires recognition of what procedures can and should be modified and what cannot or should not be, and the flexibility to make the changes mutually agreed on. As impediments to a smooth workflow are removed through cooperation, efficiency and productivity improve with a corresponding improvement to service.

Whereas cooperation removes barriers and smoothes out existing systems, collaboration generates new ideas. Raspa and Ward (2000) described collaboration as a form of creation. When people work alone they critically assess their work too quickly and do not "playfully elaborate" on an idea. In collaboration, however, ideas are more fully explored, examined, and expanded. The participants are "joined together in a relationship that brings something to life." Enterprise and innovation become possible when the diverse skills, unique strengths, and various experiences of two or more individual librarians are brought together in mutual dialogue based on common goals, trust, shared decision making, and an awareness of interdependence. Even conflict can be a form of social interaction if it is a nonemotional matter of disagreement among parties or individuals who are all working to a common goal but have different ideas of how to achieve that goal (Jones, 1997). Such constructive conflict may contribute to innovation and achievement.

BENEFITS OF SOCIAL INTERACTION
BETWEEN TECHNICAL AND PUBLIC SERVICE LIBRARIANS

If the level and quality of the social interaction between librarians, especially between the traditional divisions of public and technical services, is increased, there is a strong potential for an improvement in the work atmosphere and in the products and services the library offers to the academic community. Increased social interaction expands the opportunities for exchanging ideas, sharing knowledge and experience, and collaborating on innovative projects.

Easing or Eliminating Antagonisms Between Library Units

Technical service librarians, primarily catalogers, have been traditionally concerned with product–the creation of a catalog to the library's collection–and public service librarians, primarily reference librarians, with service–guiding patrons to the information sources they need. But product and service are not separate objectives; rather they should be recognized as two components of a single purpose. As Amy Carver (2002), a cataloger, has put it, "We are all reference librarians." There are ample accounts of the discord between what reference librarians want from the catalog and what catalogers are willing to do. From one point of view these clashes may be attributed to the catalog librarian's rigid adherence to rules and insensitivity to patron needs, and from another point of view they may be imputed to the reference librarian's disregard of essential cataloging principles and standards, and misunderstanding of the structure of a catalog record and the capabilities of the library's particular integrated library system (ILS). Or the discord could be due to a clash of the different goals and values held by catalog and reference librarians.

Through good communication, however, catalog librarians may come to understand the compelling reasons behind the reference librarians' requests for modifications or enhancements to the catalog. The reference librarians may become aware of the limitations imposed on the cataloger by the bibliographic utility the library subscribes to, the library's ILS, or by shared-catalog agreements with other libraries, and realize what the long-term impact of their requests might be on the technical services workflow and costs. As Frederick Reenstjerna (2001) pointed out, "Increased interaction between the formerly separated Reference and Technical departments is driven by the need for any library to provide a seamless access system for its clients."

Basing Decisions on the Big Picture

With an increase in social interaction between technical service and public service librarians can come an increase in the awareness of the interconnections between the various library activities. Opening reference department meetings to catalog librarians and opening technical services meetings to reference librarians is one approach to enhancing understanding and cooperation (Carver, 2002). Decisions made at integrated meetings will be more able to take into consideration the broader impact and implications to the library as a whole and will benefit from a fuller spectrum of expertise and experience. Decisions made within each department can be based on the big picture, on a real understanding of the library users' needs and the library's capabilities. As both technical service and public service librarians and staff look at a problem or situation from their different perspectives, they may be able to suggest options and alternatives that were not known to the department where the problem was identified. Decisions reached in this manner are more likely to anticipate and avoid adverse consequences, be workable within the library, and be more acceptable to everyone affected by them.

Improving Library Tools and Services

Libraries face new competitors since the new technologies have lowered the barrier to entry by commercial enterprises into the field of information providers. Libraries must find their competitive advantage or lose their hegemony (Renaud, 1997). If the library's catalog and services are to compete with Internet search engines, private companies, or even with other campus units, librarians will need to be not only responsive to their patrons' desires but also proactive in anticipating new products or services. Now that libraries face competition, librarians need to be aware of what differentiates their service from their competitors. If that distinction is quality, then they need to be sure that the quality of their product surpasses that of their competitors, or else they will lose their clients and their support.

The library's catalog is a complex structure that integrates the records for the materials in the library collection and, increasingly, for materials available electronically. The catalog librarian delineates bibliographic relationships between separate items, adds useful and consistent access points, provides sufficient information on each item for accurate identification and some pre-evaluation, correctly codes each record for effective searching in the online catalog, and maintains functional navigation between headings and cross references. "The catalog record is how we advertise to users what is available in the collection. If we do a poor job of advertising, the materials we have spent so much time, money, and effort to purchase will sit on our shelves unused" (Johnson, 1997).

To create a quality product a producer cannot work without monitoring his consumers' needs and desires and their satisfaction or dissatisfaction with the product. Yet the academic catalog librarian often works isolated from the library's patrons–the faculty and students. In order to gain that contact, some catalog librarians have found it beneficial to work shifts at the reference desk. Working side-by-side at the reference desk, technical service and public service librarians have more opportunity not only to improve the lines of communication between them but also to gain greater respect for each other and an "increased knowledge of the contributions each group makes to serving library users" (Johnson, 1997). Being able to experience for themselves the difficulties and needs of the reference staff, technical service staff may be able to propose solutions and be more willing to implement changes quickly. In addition to improving the quality of the catalog in response to their interactions with patrons, technical services librarians and staff who bring their intimate knowledge of the library's acquisitions, cataloging, and processing routines and workflow to the reference interactions may be able to enhance reference service. They may be able to search and interpret the catalog or physically locate a particular item within the library more efficiently than the reference librarians, and they can pass on some of that knowledge to the reference staff during joint shifts (Makinen, 1997).

It is not always possible or suitable that every cataloger work shifts at his library's reference desk. When this is the case, the reference librarian–as both a catalog user and a mediator between the patrons and the catalog–could be more active in improving the catalog. The reference librarian could provide the cataloger with needed feedback on the difficulties patrons encounter with the catalog or pass on the errors she encounters in the catalog during the course of duty. Additionally, with their backgrounds in various academic disciplines, reference librarians could provide the catalog librarian with invaluable help with the subject analysis of some technical materials (Intner, 1989).

As the faculty and students change their searching model to emphasize the Web and electronic resources, academic libraries need to consider redesigning their traditional reference tools to match this new model–to make "more and better resources available to our library users in the way that makes the most sense to them" (Anderson, 2002). In some libraries their web page, electronic resources, and catalog have become components of an integrated catalog, web page, or web portal.

Just as the creation of a new automobile requires the collaboration of variously skilled engineers, designers, and mechanics, so would the development of a truly useful, easily navigated, and fully integrated online tool require the diverse training, knowledge, and experience of both public service and technical service librarians.

This new integrated tool–be it a "metacatalog" (Dowlin 1991), "portal of first choice" (Binder and Yuan, 2002), "dream portal" (Jackson, 2002), or "integrated gateway" (Curtis and Greene, 2002)–could seamlessly blend the library's databases, pathfinders, bibliographies, and guides–traditionally the purview of the reference librarian–with the library's catalog–traditionally the domain of the cataloger. To this collaboration, the reference librarians, as key users of and intermediaries for this tool, would provide some of the necessary understanding of the information needs and approaches to searching of the faculty and students, apply their skills of critical selection and collection development, and would contribute some of the components in the tool. The catalogers, with their familiarity with bibliographic records and databases, of the principles and practices of organizing knowledge, and of the mechanics of the library's ILS, would create catalog records and maintain some of the links that seamlessly integrate the library's catalog with its electronic resources and its web pages.

One of the benefits of this integrated catalog may be to free the reference librarian from the confines of the physical reference desk. When the university's faculty and students are able to go to the library's catalog or portal from their own computers for many of their daily information needs instead of to the reference desk, the reference librarian gains more time for in-depth, one-on-one information consulting that incorporates instruction and research planning. Reference librarians can "move from being pointers and retrievers to facilitators and organizers. What that means in management terms is that we will have to shift our human capital investment from the end of the stream, which helps the patron find books, to the front line, which will organize information so that patrons can find it themselves" (Dowlin, 1991). A reference librarian's consulting becomes freed, by virtue of the web page, portal, or virtual library software, from the constraints of the reference desk. She is able to schedule more intensive reference consultations at a more convenient or more private location. These sessions would do more to help a harried faculty member or mystified freshman cope with the information glut they face than a fleeting encounter at the reference desk.

Collaboration Enhances the Teaching Role of Academic Libraries

The clearly defined division of responsibility has in the past usually placed bibliographic instruction to library users among the responsibilities of the reference librarians. But collaboration between catalogers and reference librarians might lead to a different approach to bibliographic instruction and information literacy, at least as it pertains to teaching faculty and students how to effectively use the library's catalog. Patricia Eskoz (1991) suggested that catalogers, who create and maintain the catalog, might be more qualified to teach searchers how to use it. By being able to teach users about the underlying structure of catalog records and the impact of that structure on searching, catalogers can help users understand the concepts involved and give them the skills to "analyze disappointing results and to explore alternative strategies" that they can apply not only to the specific setup of their library's catalog but to the different catalogs they will encounter at other libraries (Lipow, 1991).

Even if catalogers do not actively participate in bibliographic instruction to users, they must communicate to the reference staff information on changes to the catalog that come with system enhancements or migrations, or are a consequence of departmental decisions. From interaction with the catalog librarians the reference librarians will know when and how to modify their instruction to the patrons (both formal bibliographic instruction and informal reference interactions) to incorporate those changes.

Personal Benefits for Individual Librarians from Increased Social Interaction

Coping with the flood of information–journal articles, organization newsletters, topical listserves, press releases, and other information sources–can be difficult for any individual, including librarians. Through interaction with peers, a librarian may learn from a coworker of a pertinent article that he has overlooked, or hear that coworker's synopsis of an article that he has not had time to read himself. Thus through social interaction librarians can help each other to keep current on changes and issues that effect them and their work.

Communication between librarians both within a single library unit or department and between units can increase the opportunity for and encourage the development of peer and mentor relationships, and even friendships. These relationships can be of inestimable help to any librarian in the advancement of her career as well as in the enjoyment and satisfaction she derives from the work. This may also contribute significantly toward the individual's commitment to the organization and increase motivation and moral, thus possibly reducing turnover considerably (Jones, 1997; Sias and Cahill, 1998).

Avenues for Increasing Communication

Open social interaction between technical and public service librarians is the base from which improved and innovative approaches to achieving better service to the patrons can rise. Complete and timely communication is essential to promoting healthy social interaction. This means systematic and inclusive communication since, as Dixie Jones (1997) put it, "Word of mouth cannot be relied on as an effective method of spreading information." Electronic mail, with messages reaching all librarians through a group address (Jones, 1997), or a staff Intranet (Carver, 2002) are possible forms of communication that allow for cross communication and responses to the group. Regular group meetings can be an effective form of communication so long as they are run in an environment that elicits and values the concerns and suggestions of all.

The departmental policy and procedures manuals can provide another means of communication. Within the department, the manual communicates, "to each member of the team the specific behaviors that are expected and ensures that everyone is working toward the same goal" (Jones, 1997). Providing for interdepartmental access to these manuals as well would help technical service and public service librarians to understand each other.

In-house training sessions can be forums for the librarians to share their knowledge with each other and to discover each other's expertise and individual contributions toward achieving the common goal–service to the users. In addition to increasing their familiarity with each other, in-house training, as with other social interactions, may help create the synergy that leads to new ideas for better tools and services. By sharing their understanding of catalog records and the library's online catalog, catalog librarians might use an in-house training session to teach the reference librarians how to search the catalog more effectively or to introduce the reference staff to the differences in the interface of a new system. If catalog librarians attended training sessions by reference librarians they might perceive new ways to incorporate information or access into the catalog system that will help the reference staff to provide better service, or ways to more fully integrate reference databases and resources into the catalog.

A more radical approach toward increasing the interaction between technical and public services librarians would be to reorganize the library, moving away from the traditional dichotomy of functional organization to group librarians into integrated teams based on subject specialty instead. Within each team group, catalog, reference, and collection development librarians would share responsibilities in selection of materials, cataloging of those materials, and reference guidance to those materials with primary responsibility for each task falling to the appropriate individual. In this model, individual public and technical service librarians would have regular direct contact with each other. Additionally, work groups based on function (such as cataloging or reference) would provide a means for maintaining the necessary consistency in how those tasks are performed. Instead of a downwardly branching hierarchy, which may inhibit social interaction between the librarians and staff of different units, everyone would be organized into several teams that overlapped by having some common members. This structural model would increase the number of ongoing interactions between various librarians and staff. The University of Arizona's fully reorganized library structure model based on library governance groups and cross-functional teams presents a good example of increased communication in libraries in order to efficiently answer library customers' information needs (Berry, 2002).

CONCLUSION AND CELEBRATION

The ICT environment constantly creates new ways for faculty and students to search for and use information. With so many options, resources, and tools, librarians are a needed mediator in the process of accumulating knowledge. Surrounded by many commercial and campus competitors, librarians are responsible for recognizing the information needs of their faculty and students, and enhancing and developing new services and tools that would fully satisfy them. Creation of new services and tools, and enhancement of the library's catalog in order to satisfy users' information needs requires social interactions and effective communications in academic libraries.

In November 2002, the Focus on the Future Task Force of the Association of the College & Research Libraries (ACRL) released a report on the seven biggest issues facing academic libraries. Those issues are:

1. Recruitment, education, and retention of librarians;
2. Role of library in academic enterprise;
3. Impact of information technology on library services;
4. Creation, control, and preservation of digital resources;
5. Chaos in scholarly communication;
6. Support of new users;
7. Higher education funding (Hisle, 2002).

Librarians are aware of these issues. Finding answers to all of them are important for the future of academic libraries but this report omitted two crucial issues–change of organizational structure and effective assessment of library services. In the last five years, much has been written on adjusting academic libraries to technological changes (Schwartz, 1997), new academic library models (Rader, 2001), and college libraries in a new age (Morris, 2002). In the reviewed literature on academic libraries two common calls are strong and clear–a call for organizational change and a call for assessment of library services. Neither of these issues is addressed by the ACRL report. As Carla Stoffle stated, "Libraries have to change, and the driver for change is economics. It is not technology–technology can be an enabler if we use it right–but . . . we simply cannot afford to keep doing things the same old way" (Berry, 2002). The old organizational model, with its separate departments for public and technical services, and its hierarchical routes of communication, inhibits social interaction between librarians and makes communication within the library inefficient. Lack of efficient social interaction and communication between librarians slows academic libraries as an effective provider of quality services to the academic community. Social interaction and good communication does matter. It contributes to the decision-making process, mitigates interpersonal and interdepartmental conflicts, increases staff moral and camaraderie, encourages collaboration, fosters innovation, and expands opportunities. Most importantly it improves service and teaching.

REFERENCES

Anderson, Rick (2002), [Letter to the editor], *The Chronicle of Higher Education* (July 26), B18.
Berry, John, N. (2002), "Arizona's New Model," *Library Journal* 127 (November 1), 40-42.
Binder, Michael B. and Yuan, Haiwang (2002), "TIP–The Web-Based Library Portal at Western Kentucky University and Its Implications for Libraries Becoming 'Portals of First Choice' for Their Communities," *Technical Services Quarterly* 19 (4), 1-15.

Blurton, Craig (1999), "New Direction in Education," in *World Communication and Information Report 1999-2000*. Paris: UNESCO, 46-61.

Budd, John M. (1998), *The Academic Library: Its Context, Its Purpose, and Its Operation*. Englewood, Colo.: Libraries Unlimited.

Carlson, Scott (2002), "Students and Faculty Members Turn to Online Library Materials Before Printed Ones, Study Finds," *Chronicle of Higher Education* (October 3). Retrieved November 14, 2002, from http://chronicle.com/free/2002/10/2002100301t.htm.

Carver, Amy L. (2002), "We Are All Reference Librarians: Using Communication to Employ a Philosophy of Access for Catalogers," *College & Research Libraries News* 63 (March), 168-170.

Curtis, Donnelyn and Greene, Araby Y. (2002), "Presenting the Virtual Library," in *Attracting, Educating, and Serving Remote Users Through the Web*, edited by Donnelyn Curtis. New York: Neal-Shuman, 39-71.

Dowlin, Kenneth E. (1991), "Public Libraries in 2001," *Information Technology and Libraries* 10 (December), 317-321.

Eskoz, Patricia A. (1991), "Catalog Librarians and Public Services–A Changing Role?" *Library Resources & Technical Services* 35 (1), 76-86.

Hisle, W. Lee (2002), "Top Issues Facing Academic Libraries: A Report of the Focus on the Future Task Force," *College & Research Libraries News* 63 (November). Retrieved November 14, 2002, from http://www.ala.org/acrl/hislenov02.html.

Intner, Sheila (1989), "Ten Good Reasons Why Reference Librarians Would Make Good Catalogers," *Technicalities* 9 (January), 14-16.

Jackson, Mary E. (2002), "The Advent of Portals," *Library Journal*, (September 15), 36-39.

Jankowska, Maria Anna (2003), "Economic Aspects of Recorded Knowledge" in *Encyclopedia of Library and Information Science*. New York: Marcel Dekker, Vol. 2, p. 944-950.

Johnson, Bonnie E. (1997), "Crossing the Line: A Cataloger Goes Public," in *Philosophies of Reference*, edited by Celia Hales Mabry. New York: The Haworth Press, Inc., 147-151.

Jones, Dixie A. (1997), "Plays Well with Others, or the Importance of Collegiality Within a Reference Unit," in *Philosophies of Reference*, edited by Celia Hales Mabry. New York: The Haworth Press, Inc., 163-175.

Lipow, Anne G. (1991), "Teach Online Catalog Users the MARC Format? Are You Kidding?" *Journal of Academic Librarianship* 17 (May). Retrieved September 24, 2002, from EBSCO database (MasterFILE Premier) on the World Wide Web.

Makinen, Ruth H. (1997), "Scheduling Technical Services Staff at the Reference Desk," in *Philosophies of Reference*, edited by Celia Hales Mabry. New York: The Haworth Press, Inc., 139-146.

Mansell, Robin (1996), "Communication by Design?" in *Communication by Design: The Politics of Information and Communication Technologies*, edited by Robin Mansell and Roger Silverston. New York: Oxford University Press, 15-43.

Morris, Jeff (2002), "The College Library in the New Age," *University Business* (October). Retrieved Nov. 14, 2002, from http://www.universitybusiness.com/story.asp?txtFilename=features/library.htm.

Rader, Hannelore B. (2001), "A New Academic Library Model: Partnership for Learning and Teaching," *College and Research Libraries News* 62 (April). Retrieved November 18, 2002, from http://www.ala.org/acrl/rader.html.

Raspa, Dick and Dane Ward (2000), "Listening for Collaboration: Faculty and Librarians Working Together," in *The Collaborative Imperative: Librarians and Faculty Working Together in the Information Universe*, edited by Dick Raspa and Dane Ward. Chicago: Association of College and Research Libraries, 1-18.

Reenstjerna, Frederick (2001), "Thinking About Reference Service Paradigms and Metaphors," in *Doing the Work of Reference: Practical Tips for Excelling as a Reference Librarian*, edited by Celia Hales Mabry. New York: The Haworth Press, Inc., 97-111.

Renaud, Robert (1997), "Learning to Compete: Competition, Outsourcing, and Academic Libraries," *Journal of Academic Librarianship* 23 (March), 85-90.

Rummel, R. J. (1976), *Understanding Conflict and War, vol. 2, The Conflict Helix.* New York: John Wiley & Sons.

Schwartz, Charles, A. (1997), "Reconstructing Academic Libraries: Adjusting to Technological Change," in *Restructuring Academic Libraries: Organizational Development in the Wake of Technological Change*, edited by Charles A. Schwartz. Chicago: Association of College and Research Libraries, 1-30.

Sias, Patricia M. and Cahill, Daniel J. (1998), "From Coworkers to Friends: The Development of Peer Friendships in the Workplace," *Western Journal of Communication* 62 (3), 273+. Retrieved September 24, 2002, from EBSCO database (MasterFILE Premier) on the World Wide Web.

Cooperative Reference and Collection Development: The Science and Technology Group at the University of Tennessee Libraries

Teresa U. Berry
Flora G. Shrode

SUMMARY. The science and technology subject group within the reference department of the University of Tennessee Libraries brings together librarians from reference and other departments who have collection development and subject liaison duties. The authors describe the group's composition and explain how the sci/tech librarians work cooperatively toward goals set by both the Libraries' Reference & Instructional Services and Collection Development & Management departments. The sci/tech group's primary cooperative functions are to facilitate librarians' mutual assistance in organizing projects, share insights for reference and collection development/management activities, plan instruction efforts, discuss web site development, promote mastery of resources and tools, and address other concerns. The subject group en-

Teresa U. Berry is Science Librarian, University of Tennessee Libraries, 1015 Volunteer Boulevard, Knoxville, TN 37922-1000 (E-mail: berry@aztec.lib.utk.edu). Flora G. Shrode is Interim Head of Reference Services, Utah State University Libraries, Logan, UT 84322 (E-mail: fshrode@cc.usu.edu).

[Haworth co-indexing entry note]: "Cooperative Reference and Collection Development: The Science and Technology Group at the University of Tennessee Libraries." Berry, Teresa U., and Flora G. Shrode. Co-published simultaneously in *The Reference Librarian* (The Haworth Information Press, an imprint of The Haworth Press, Inc.) No. 83/84, 2003, pp. 145-155; and: *Cooperative Reference: Social Interaction in the Workplace* (ed: Celia Hales Mabry) The Haworth Information Press, an imprint of The Haworth Press, Inc., 2003, pp. 145-155. Single or multiple copies of this article are available for a fee from The Haworth Document Delivery Service [1-800-HAWORTH, 9:00 a.m. - 5:00 p.m. (EST). E-mail address: docdelivery@haworthpress.com].

http://www.haworthpress.com/web/REF
Digital Object Identifier: 10.1300J120v40n83_12

ables librarians to clarify plans and procedures and to come to grips with complicated budget matters. A fundamental benefit of group discussions is that they provide an opportunity to explore viewpoints from librarians outside the reference team, leading to more well-rounded decisions. Together with the other subject groups, the sci/tech librarians and their coordinator identify major needs for information and work to provide solutions that improve library services to the academic community. *[Article copies available for a fee from The Haworth Document Delivery Service: 1-800-HAWORTH. E-mail address: <docdelivery@haworthpress.com> Website: <http://www.HaworthPress.com> © 2003 by The Haworth Press, Inc. All rights reserved.]*

KEYWORDS. Interprofessional cooperation, reference department organization, reference services organization, collection development management, subject librarians

INTRODUCTION

There is no question that computer technology, particularly the World Wide Web, has had a tremendous impact on academic libraries. Not only did information technology dramatically change users' access to library collections and services, but it also had a profound effect in the library workplace. The growing emphasis in collection development on electronic resources altered the library's organizational dynamics and increased the level of interdepartmental cooperation. Many collection development and management activities that were once the sole responsibility of a single department are now shared in ways that have led to new organizational models (Webb, 2001). Driven by increasing user demand and escalating costs for electronic full-text resources, libraries are increasingly turning to cooperative collection development agreements and other creative financial arrangements.

The pervasive use of technology has also changed the nature of library jobs, shifting from traditional, functional specialist positions to more expansive and complex jobs (Lynch and Smith, 2001). The information age, characterized by increasing dependence on the Web for information, reshaped the roles and responsibilities of reference librarians. Although members of the Association of Research Libraries (ARL) reported a decline in reference transactions during the past ten years, Jackson reports that reference librarians' workloads are expanding tremendously to include more collection development and liaison responsibilities (Jackson, 2002). Reference departments have often added new services and outreach initiatives without adding more personnel.

The collaborative environment within the reference department at the University of Tennessee Libraries is key to its success as a service-oriented organization. Cooperative efforts make many reference services and outreach initiatives possible at the University of Tennessee Libraries. This paper focuses on the role of the Science/Technology group, one of the subject groups in the organizational structure of Reference & Instructional Services (RIS) and Collection Development & Management (CDM) departments. The science librarians work with the other subject librarians and collaborate with personnel from other departments to extend information services and resources to the university campus and to participate in consortium partnerships with other libraries.

THE REFERENCE DEPARTMENT

When the John C. Hodges Library opened its doors in 1987, the services and collections of the Undergraduate Library and the James D. Hoskins Main Library were consolidated in a single building. To cope with the managerial responsibilities of a department that suddenly doubled in size, the head of reference adopted an organization scheme to distribute some of the supervisory responsibilities among three newly created subject coordinator positions. Reference librarians were assigned to one of three subject groups according to their strengths and interests: arts and humanities, social sciences, and science and technology (sci/tech). Although some aspects of the original organizational structure, particularly those associated with functional positions, changed over the years, the subject groups remained a constant force within the department. Today the Reference & Instructional Services Department (RIS) at the University of Tennessee Libraries has twenty-two faculty and 8.5 FTE staff. The department head supervises eight librarians (Figure 1) as well as two FTE. The remaining thirteen reference librarians belong to a subject group and are directly supervised by a subject coordinator.

The three subject coordinators are unique in that they report to both the head of RIS and the head of Collection Development & Management (CDM). The subject coordinators direct the reference and collection development activities of their respective groups,

FIGURE 1. UT Libraries Reference Department Organization

```
┌─────────────────────────────────┐
│ Head, Reference Department       │
└─────────────────────────────────┘
    │
    ├──────┌─────────────────────────────────────────────────┐
    │      │              Humanities Coordinator*             │
    │      └─────────────────────────────────────────────────┘
    │            ┌──────────────────────────────────┐
    │            │          4 Librarians             │
    │            └──────────────────────────────────┘
    ├──────┌─────────────────────────────────────────────────┐
    │      │          Science/Technology Coordinator*         │
    │      └─────────────────────────────────────────────────┘
    │            ┌──────────────────────────────────┐
    │            │          4 Librarians             │
    │            └──────────────────────────────────┘
    ├──────┌─────────────────────────────────────────────────┐
    │      │           Social Sciences Coordinator*           │
    │      └─────────────────────────────────────────────────┘
    │            ┌──────────────────────────────────┐
    │            │          5 Librarians             │
    │            └──────────────────────────────────┘
    ├──────┌─────────────────────────────────────────────────┐
    │      │          Distance Education Librarian            │
    │      └─────────────────────────────────────────────────┘
    ├──────┌─────────────────────────────────────────────────┐
    │      │         Electronic Services Coordinator*         │
    │      └─────────────────────────────────────────────────┘
    ├──────┌─────────────────────────────────────────────────┐
    │      │   Government Documents/Microforms Coordinator    │
    │      └─────────────────────────────────────────────────┘
    ├──────┌─────────────────────────────────────────────────┐
    │      │         Instructional Services Coordinator       │
    │      └─────────────────────────────────────────────────┘
    └──────┌─────────────────────────────────────────────────┐
           │                  Map Librarian                   │
           └─────────────────────────────────────────────────┘
```

*Also reports to Head, Collection Development and Management.

oversee collection development budget allocations and expenditures for their areas, provide reference and instruction, serve as subject liaison for selected departments, and supervise the main library's reference librarians with the group. The head of RIS holds regular meetings with the subject and the other coordinators to address departmental management concerns, plan programs, and organize projects at both the departmental and library-wide levels. A standing committee known as the Collection Development & Management Advisory Group oversees collection development and management activities. The head of the CDM department chairs the advisory group and convenes weekly meetings; its membership includes the subject coordinators, the head of reference, the CDM coordinator, the preservation librarian, a representative from the four branch libraries, and the head of technical services who supervises cataloging and acquisitions. This group's broad representation facilitates communication from many directions since librarians on the advisory group solicit feedback from all parts of the organization, and they can also enlist additional personnel with appropriate skills and expertise to help accomplish objectives.

With the exception of the instruction coordinator and electronic services coordinator, each reference librarian also has collection development and management responsibilities for assigned subject areas, serving as liaison to one or more academic departments. Liaison assignments are determined by attempting to match campus and library needs to the librarian's educational background and prior job experience. The subject coordinators and the heads of RIS and CDM work together to distribute the liaison workloads equitably, recognizing that academic departments vary in their demands for attention and interaction. The subject assignments, however, can change in response to internal and external factors. For example, job turnover can cause subject coordinators to reassign liaison duties until a new librarian is hired, a process that can span several months. These temporary rearrangements are necessary so that reference and instructional services for the affected faculty and students are not disrupted. Changes in the university's organization, such as the merging or disbanding of academic departments, can also force the coordinators to examine the assignments.

Although the subject groups were originally envisioned as subunits of the Reference Department, they have become a mechanism for encouraging librarians from other library departments to participate in collection development activities. These individuals either volunteer or are recruited to be subject librarians because of expertise developed through past education or prior job experience. The term "subject librarian" does not serve as the individual's job title, but instead refers to that person's additional role as a liaison to a particular academic department. As of August 2002, eleven of the twenty-eight subject librarians are from departments outside of Reference. Most often they have responsibility for collection development and management but do not provide instruction, although they may collaborate with reference librarians to plan or teach classes cooperatively. These hybrid assignments create "opportunities for collaboration, for the use of expertise, and for discovering affinities among functions that are not reflected in the functional organization" (Eckwright and Bolin, 2001).

THE SCIENCE/TECHNOLOGY GROUP

The science/technology group is comprised of eleven subject librarians from several areas of the library: reference, technical services, the business office, and two branch libraries (Table 1). The sci/tech coordinator and four reference librarians are gathered administratively in the reference department of Hodges Library. The remaining members of the group include a cataloger (who is now the serials librarian), the Libraries' business manager, the map librarian, and three branch librari-

TABLE 1. The Science/Technology Group

Position	Subject Areas
Sci/Tech Coordinator	Biochemistry, Cellular & Molecular Biology
Reference Librarian	Botany Ecology & Environmental Biology Microbiology
Reference Librarian	Chemistry Computer Science Physics
Reference Librarian	Engineering Textiles
Reference Librarian	Audiology & Speech Pathology Health, Safety & Exercise Sciences Nursing Nutrition
Map Librarian	Geography
Head, Agriculture-Veterinary Medicine Library	Agricultural Sciences & Natural Resources Latin American Studies Portuguese, Spanish
Reference Librarian, Agriculture-Veterinary Medicine Library	Agricultural Sciences & Natural Resources
Reference Librarian, Agriculture-Veterinary Medicine Library	Veterinary Medicine
Business Manager	Mathematics Information Sciences
Serials Librarian	Geology

ans from the Agriculture-Veterinary Medicine Library. Two sci/tech subject librarians also belong to other subject groups by virtue of having liaison responsibilities for areas in the social sciences and humanities.

The sci/tech group meets at least once a month to discuss library and campus issues, but the primary focus is on collection development and management. Although the librarians represent the interests of their respective subject areas, they must work together to make the best decisions that meet the needs of the university. The boundaries that delineated the subject areas in the past are blurring as researchers collaborate across disciplines and academic departments. Not only are new disciplines created, but the traditional subjects are also changed or "hybridized" (Pugh, 1995). The sci/tech librarians are careful to consult with one another to assess the impact of collection development decisions, such as canceling a journal subscription or changing database vendors, and try to ensure that "loyalty to a specific library or audience must be balanced against the needs of interdisciplinary users" (Wilson & Edelman, 1996).

Collection development discussions are not necessarily limited to science and technology areas. Ever mindful of the fact that sci/tech has a large share of the budget, the sci/tech group weighs the needs of the humanities and social sciences and makes recommendations that benefit the campus as a whole. For example, each subject group compiles a ranked list of desired databases, journals, large microfiche collections, and other expensive items. The sci/tech group then looks at the humanities and social sciences lists and gives the coordinator feedback on where the sci/tech priorities fit within the larger wish list. The sci/tech coordinator takes the group's opinions back to the CDM Advisory Group, which can then reach a consensus on what is the best course of action.

No separate science and engineering library exists on the main campus, so the four sci/tech reference librarians share the responsibility of providing reference services in the main library where they encounter many types of users, such as a freshman English student looking for literary criticism or a businessman from the community needing industry ratios. The wide variety of questions requires the sci/tech librarian to be familiar with information resources in many disciplines, including the humanities and social sciences. Up to three librarians are scheduled for reference desk duty during the day when classes are in session, thus providing an opportunity for sci/tech librarians to interact with librarians from other subject groups. One of the benefits of such an arrangement is that the librarians can take advantage of their colleagues' knowledge and expertise and learn about new resources or search techniques in an immediate practical situation. The sci/tech librarians will also help staff the reference desk at the Agriculture-Veterinary Medicine Library when there is a staffing shortage or when the branch staff attends their annual planning retreat. The sci/tech librarians at UT find that this diversity at the reference desk plays an important role in job satisfaction.

The sci/tech reference librarians also work closely with their reference colleagues on projects and initiatives that contribute to the goals and mission of the reference department as well as perform functions that are integral to departmental operations. The head of RIS convenes departmental task forces and ad hoc committees that have representatives from each of the three subject groups; thus, librarians from humanities, sciences, and social sciences can bring the different perspectives of their constituencies into the planning and implementation of services. These subgroups may have short-term projects, such as redesigning the physical layout of the reference room or creating web pages that serve as virtual business cards for all the subject librarians. They can also have long-term responsibilities, such as maintaining the reference web site and coordinating digital reference services. The sci/tech librarians also collaborate with the instructional coordinator in developing online tutorials for freshman English students and other information literacy initiatives.

COOPERATION WITH OTHER LIBRARIES

UT Libraries maintains a close relationship with the Preston Medical Library at the University of Tennessee Medical Center, which is located within a mile of the Knoxville campus. Although the Medical Center is administratively tied to the University of Tennessee at Memphis, UT Libraries provides cataloging and document delivery services for Preston. The collaboration has also promoted resource sharing, especially among nursing and veterinary medicine faculty and students who often need access to specialized medical titles available at the hospital library. In return, the broader collection of materials at UT Libraries complements the size and budget of the smaller library. The staffs at both libraries share the same high standards for service and are comfortable encouraging users to use the other library.

Electronic editions of journals have proven especially helpful for the hospital library both for ease of access and reduced need for space to house print collections. The electronic services coordinator, serials librarian, and head of UT Libraries' CDM department collaborated to establish methods for sharing costs and stipulating terms of access in licenses for online products. For example, some researchers who work at UT Hospital have joint appointments with academic departments in the university, primarily in biological science departments such as microbiology and biochemistry; thus, they count as part of the campus's FTE used in the formula to set subscription prices. The researchers were initially blocked from accessing e-journals because the IP addresses associated with the hospital offices and laboratories do not fall within the range provided in the licensing agreements. Since Preston Library shares the catalog with UT Libraries, researchers were often confused when they wanted to view electronic journals from UT Libraries' collections but were denied access from their hospital offices and laboratories. UT science librarians worked with the electronic services coordinator and hospital library staff to resolve problems by creating a separate user authentication system. In their capacity as UT faculty, these researchers may have individual accounts similar to distance education students so that they may view electronic journals and databases, bypassing access restrictions controlled by IP address.

Cooperation with other institutions also occurs through a consortium called the Information Alliance, which has three member libraries: University of Tennessee, University of Kentucky, and Vanderbilt University. "With the advent of new technologies, the rise of consortia with shared resources, and the availability of multiple document delivery options, libraries have shifted from a classical collection development model of material ownership to an eclectic model of providing timely access to materials" (Frank et al., 1999). A goal of the Information Alliance is that "the holdings of the three libraries be used by patrons at the three institutions as if they were one collection" (Information Alliance). A common catalog was developed, and arrangements were made for expedited interlibrary loans. Subject librarians from UT meet with their counterparts from Kentucky and Vanderbilt to discuss collection development issues and to explore collaborative efforts. Discussion topics in the past included identifying subject areas where a single library would be the primary collector for highly specialized materials and cooperatively archiving little used books and journals. The Information Alliance has also been able to make joint purchases of bibliographic and full-text databases.

COOPERATION WITH OTHER CAMPUS UNITS

Reference librarians are leaders in forming partnerships with campus groups and setting the tone for the Libraries' relations with the university. The sci/tech subject coordinator served as a non-voting member on the natural sciences division of the College of Arts & Sciences' curriculum committee that represents the broad disciplinary divisions of science. This affords the Libraries an opportunity to learn about changes in teaching emphases, so they can purchase necessary materials or be prepared to support specific needs of large populations of students in service courses. The electronic services coordinator served as co-chair of the Research Council, a Faculty Senate sub-group charged with tracking policies and procedures governing the university's research programs. While serving in that post, this librarian helped to establish a faculty computer equipment refresh program that oversees distribution of university computer services funding to buy faculty members upgrades for their computer equipment on a three-year cycle. Another librarian serves on the Teaching Council, the Faculty Senate sub-group that advocates for standards, infrastructure, and overall needs required for high quality instruction.

Librarians have worked to make their services visible through the university's course management software (CMS) system to provide a visible link to the digital reference service *AskUs.Now!* from the university's portal, Online@UT, that uses the Blackboard software. The Innovative Technology Center (ITC) supports online courses and manages UT's implementation of the Blackboard software. Since its introduction on the UT campus, the Libraries' distance education librarian uses Blackboard both to teach sessions with students from a variety of classes and as a means to communicate with geographically remote students, offering them assistance with all aspects of research and obtaining library materials. Her expertise has helped reference librarians understand the system, so they can help students who come to the Libraries to access their course materials. In 2001/2002 reference librarians worked in cooperation with the Innovative Technologies Center staff for training to achieve CMS certification. Reference librarians have created a "Library Resources" module that links to key library information. A Blackboard working group has emerged, led by the social sciences reference coordinator, and they have established web links from Online@UT to library tutorials and subject guides. The electronic services coordinator has worked with ITC to create an instructional web site to provide professors with guidance about how to incorporate online library resources into web tools they develop for their classes.

CONCLUSION

The role of the subject librarian in collection development is changing as libraries turn their attention on the acquisition of large, multidisciplinary periodical collections such as ScienceDirect and ProQuest. The nature of the licensing and/or agreements with consortia often take some of the decision-making out of the subject librarian's hands (Welch, 2002).

The sci/tech subject group in the University of Tennessee Libraries provides some structure for its members in a work environment where change is constant and many needs compete for their time and attention.

Within the group librarians can float ideas, get help when workloads peak, and organize effort toward meeting objectives set by the Reference Team and other Libraries task forces. Without formal goals or policies, the group is project-oriented and contributes to activities initiated from other parts of the Libraries and, occasionally, from outside the library. Subject groups are logical for UT Libraries' reference department because of its size. In light of the broad range of responsibilities in subject librarians' jobs, this organizational model allows for flexibility and responsiveness, takes advantage of individual talents, and fosters learning and development.

REFERENCES

Eckwright, Gail Z. and Bolin, Mary K. (2001),"The Hybrid Librarian: The Affinity of Collection Management with Technical Services and the Organizational Benefits of an Individualized Assignment," *Journal of Academic Librarianship* 27 (November), 452-456.

Information Alliance, University of Tennessee, Vanderbilt University, and University of Kentucky: Counterpart Projects (n.d.). Retrieved January 16, 2003, from http://www.lib.utk.edu/~alliance/counterpartprojects.html.

Jackson, Rebecca (2002), "Revolution or Evolution: Reference Planning in ARL Libraries," *Reference Services Review* 30 (3), 212-228.

Lynch, Beverly P. and Smith, Kimberley Robles (2001), "The Changing Nature of Work in Academic Libraries," *College & Research Libraries* 62 (September), 407-420.

Pugh, Stephen (1995), "When Selectors Collide: The Challenge of Interdisciplinary Scholarship for Collection Development: A Panel Discussion," *Library Acquisitions: Practice & Theory* 20 (Summer), 187-190.

Webb, John (2001), "Collections and Systems: A New Organizational Paradigm for Collection Development," *Library Collections, Acquisitions, & Technical Services* 25 (Winter), 461-468.

Welch, Jeanie M. (2002), "Hey! What About Us?! Changing Roles of Subject Specialists and Reference Librarians in the Age of Electronic Resources," *Serials Review* 28 (Winter), 283-286.

Wilson, Myoung Chung and Edelman, Hendrik (1996), "Collection Development in an Interdisciplinary Context," *Journal of Academic Librarianship* 22 (May), 195-200.

Improving Reference Services
Through a Library Website:
Strategies for Collaborative Change

Debra Engel
Sarah Robbins

SUMMARY. Websites are virtual front doors to the university library for many distance education students and for those simply choosing to access the numerous resources available to them through the library from off-campus. A driving force behind the redesign of the library website was to provide a user-friendly, content-rich website that offers assistance at the point of need, wherever the student is located. The University of Oklahoma Libraries' Web Committee's research and develop-

Debra Engel (E-mail: dhengel@ou.edu) is Director of Public Services and Sarah Robbins (E-mail: srobbins@ou.edu) is Electronic Services Coordinator, both at University Libraries, University of Oklahoma, 401 West Brooks, Norman, OK 73019.

[Haworth co-indexing entry note]: "Improving Reference Services Through a Library Website: Strategies for Collaborative Change." Engel, Debra, and Sarah Robbins. Co-published simultaneously in *The Reference Librarian* (The Haworth Information Press, an imprint of The Haworth Press, Inc.) No. 83/84. 2003, pp. 157-173; and: *Cooperative Reference: Social Interaction in the Workplace* (ed: Celia Hales Mabry) The Haworth Information Press, an imprint of The Haworth Press, Inc., 2003, pp. 157-173. Single or multiple copies of this article are available for a fee from The Haworth Document Delivery Service [1-800-HAWORTH. 9:00 a.m. - 5:00 p.m. (EST). E-mail address: docdelivery@haworthpress.com].

Digital Object Identifier: 10.1300J120v40n83_13   *157*

ment focus combined with a collaborative environment provided a positive impetus for change to the library website and improved reference services to the University community. *[Article copies available for a fee from The Haworth Document Delivery Service: 1-800-HAWORTH. E-mail address: <docdelivery@haworthpress.com> Website: <http://www.HaworthPress.com> © 2003 by The Haworth Press, Inc. All rights reserved.]*

KEYWORDS. Collaboration, website design, reference services, academic libraries

Academic library reference services have changed dramatically in recent years as a result of increased access to electronic resources. Traditionally, the library's reference desk was the starting point for research assistance for many library users; however, the library website is fast becoming the primary point of contact with the library for many students and researchers. Websites are virtual front doors to the library for distance education students and for those simply choosing to access the numerous library resources available to them through the library from off-campus. Sadly enough, the harsh reality is that some students may seldom, if ever, enter the library during their tenure at the university. To meet customer demands, libraries must evaluate how they present themselves to the world through their library's website.

Revising the University of Oklahoma Libraries website (http://libraries. ou.edu) offered the library an opportunity to provide more effective reference services for students and faculty. Providing a user-friendly, content-rich website that offers assistance at the point of need wherever the student is located was a driving force behind the redesign of the library website. The effective library website brings together all of the library's resources, print and electronic. It offers guidance while fostering independent learning. University Libraries created a Web Committee charged with improving the effectiveness of the library's website through more consistent navigation, a more intuitive design, and added content. The University of Oklahoma Web Committee utilized a collaborative group process that provided a forum for problem-solving through research to develop a new library web interface for the campus community. This paper investigates the collaborative process utilized by the Web Committee and discusses the organization's cultural dynamics that influenced decisions and interactions among group members.

BACKGROUND

In the fall of 2001 the University Libraries' staff and administration felt that a change was needed in the library website in order to better meet the needs of the students and faculty. The previous Web Committee had met over a two-year period and suggested possible standards for the website; however, few changes were made to the structure and the suggested standards were not enforced. A new Web Committee was formed and chaired by the Director of Public Services. The committee charge from the University Libraries' Dean was two-part: to provide the research and development testing ground for a unified web interface for the website and to provide improved and consistent navigation within the library website. Guidelines suggested at the University of Alberta Libraries in regard to teamwork state that successful teams "start with a clear mandate. A mandate describes what question needs answering, what perceived problem needs to be dealt with and/or what process needs to be reviewed and improved" (Soete, 1998). The Dean's charge provided the Web Committee with the focus it needed to succeed. The Dean also requested a short implementation schedule with results expected by January 2002.

The primary purpose of the library website is to provide a virtual front door for the resources of University Libraries. The shared vision developed by the Web Committee during the course of the semester was that the website should be a "one-stop shop" for the student with a research need and provide a starting place for assignments for both undergraduate and graduate students. As Stover notes, "The academic library Web site can support research in higher education through providing access to Internet research tools and full-text databases. It can support teaching through online full-text reserves and other means. And it can support public service through allowing the general public (and other libraries) to access its online resources, including the online public access catalog" (1997).

Members of the Web Committee felt an obligation to produce timely and effective results. The environment within University Libraries was that something had to be done about the library website. One underlying motivation shared by the committee members was that there was a need for change in the library website in order to provide subject access to resources and a more consistent navigation scheme. Although there were no visible accomplishments as a result of the work of the first Web Committee, such as changes to the website, the background work of the former committee proved useful by giving the new committee a foundation upon which to build. The initial Web Committee established guide-lines for those wishing to publish on the library website and had spent a considerable amount of time analyzing the websites of other libraries. Since some members of the initial Web Committee were on the newly created Web Committee, this knowledge and previous work was able to be shared with the new members.

BUILDING A CULTURE OF COLLABORATION

The Web Committee was composed of seventeen faculty and staff members from a cross-section of University Libraries including public services, technical services, systems, and administration. Diversity of representation served to make the committee stronger than it would have been had the committee been composed of only members from a few departments or specializations. As Bunker and Zick assert, "The required synergy can only come from bringing together people with the appropriate skills and vision. Each must comprehend and embrace diverse roles in learning and the application of learning to the creation of new knowledge" (1999). The chair set the stage at the first group meeting that defined the purpose of the website, the objectives of the Web Committee (with deadlines), the ground rules for the operation, and the concept of breaking into work groups to accomplish the variety of tasks necessary to fulfill the objectives. The chair of the Web Committee had been with University Libraries for less than one year, which had both advantages and disadvantages. The chair did not have a history with the existing organizational culture. One of the first tasks of the committee chair was to provide a collaborative environment where the individual group members felt that they could trust each other and the process in a new entrepreneurial venture. As Dupuis and Ryan write of their experiences with collaboration, "Without a commitment to compromise, we would be constantly in danger of deadlocking on important decisions" (2002). The previous Web Committee had difficulty producing results because of endless discussions that were never resolved. To prevent the same scenario in the new Web Committee, the chair encouraged discussion with an expectation of decisions and action plans that best served the overall Web Committee mission.

Brainstorming ground rules at the first meeting was important to the group process utilized by the Web Committee and one of the features that distinguished the Web Committee from other library committees.

To function effectively and efficiently a team needs operating ground rules. These are set by the team itself as internal "rules of conduct." Ground rules are oriented towards team performance and goal achievement and help to foster openness, trust and commitment. The rules may pertain to attendance, confidentiality, how the team will conduct its meetings, definition of consensus (e.g., is silence agreement?), and members' contributions. Ground rules must be followed and enforced. (Soete, 1997)

Ground rules encompassed expectations of the logistics of meeting management as well as behaviors expected of committee members such as no tolerance for attacks on individuals. Using the staff intranet as a means of communication between meetings was encouraged. In addition, ground rules provided an operational framework for civil discourse. The chair also asked members to submit possible mission statements for the website prior to the first meeting based on the University Libraries' mission and vision statements. These were discussed at the first meeting and a mission statement for the library website was decided: "To inform the campus community about the resources and services of University Libraries within a user-friendly, intuitive navigation style."

The group process that evolved was one of testing assumptions and expectations and providing a safe arena for exploring new ideas and concepts. The learning curve for many committee members was high. Public and technical services employees had to learn the principles of good web design while systems office staff had to learn about library operations. In order to improve services via the website there were several discussions about how to best serve undergraduate students with vague assignments, how to serve students who had little knowledge about databases and ejournals, and how to serve graduate students and faculty with advanced research needs.

Creating a collaborative culture of learning and testing ideas was relatively new to the organizational culture of University Libraries. Not everyone on the Web Committee was comfortable with the idea that individuals could agree to disagree about an issue. It took several weeks of meetings before Web Committee members were able to understand the diversity of the Web Committee and appreciate each other's strengths and talents. One of the jobs of the committee chair was to provide a consistent vision of the Web Committee's objectives and reinforce that vision through communication, enthusiasm, and commitment. The chair was dedicated to creating a collaborative climate that embraced inclusiveness of ideas and helped committee members learn to appreciate diverse thinking.

THE ROLE OF WORK GROUPS

Each Web Committee member was expected to serve on a work group. The work groups took large objectives and broke the tasks into manageable parts. The work group structure had not been used in previous university library committees. Some work groups were more effective in accomplishing their assigned tasks than others. Nevertheless, the work groups were an essential part of the Web Committee environment and crucial to the success or failure of the effort. The work groups played an important role in the marketing of the new website to colleagues within the library as well as across campus. Web Committee members were able to return to their respective departments and publicize the latest developments of the committee as well as solicit feedback from their colleagues. Manning notes that "customer obsession begins and ends with relationships. Web teams are no longer managing projects, they are managing relationships" (2002). By getting feedback from library colleagues and from departmental liaisons across campus, the Web Committee utilized their relationships in these areas to improve the website and, thus, improve customer service by giving the customers what they wanted and not just giving them what the committee thought they wanted.

Three work groups were established at the initial Web Committee meeting. These work groups were responsible for visual design, web content, and subject access to electronic resources. Each work group was composed of personnel from public services, technical services and systems. As Smith, Tedford, and Womack state, "When all areas of a library are represented on a team, there are increased feelings of ownership by the entire organization" (2001). Every area had a voice in each work group so all needs could be represented and taken into consideration before final decisions were made. A chair for each work group was nominated during the first Web Committee meeting.

Visual Design Work Group. The visual design work group was charged with developing a unified look for the website that incorporated consistent navigational tools for use on every page within the website. To do this effectively, the work group examined a large number of other library websites to compare navigation schemes and looked at logical relationships between content already on the site and content that would be added to create a coherent hierarchy for display of the information. The goal was to design the site so that users would intuitively know where to look for the information on the site with a minimal number of clicks and with little outside instruction. McMullen explains, "The library Web interface represents a critical meeting ground between the information professional and the individual who is seeking information. . . . The Web interface should be clear and uncluttered, easy to maneuver, and provide built-in redundancy to accommodate different learning styles" (2001). The visual design work group reviewed many different color schemes and fonts so that the look and feel of the site would present a positive image of University Libraries. The chair of the Web Committee took the group's recommendations to the Dean of University Libraries so he could voice his opinion and provide feedback to the group. This was an important intervention because it gave the group permission to move forward and discuss other issues. The visual design work group also considered the newly developed university-wide ADA (Americans with Disabilities Act) standards for websites that were implemented during the semester.

Content Work Group. The content work group was given the task of reviewing the content currently on the library website and suggesting which content would make the migration to the new site as well as suggesting what new content would be developed for the new site. It was quickly realized by those on this work group that separating content from visual design may not have been as logical as it had originally seemed. Since content and design are closely connected and drive one another, it was difficult for the content work group to make many decisions that would not affect visual design and vice versa. In an article discussing the process of creating a University website at Oregon State University, Davidson and Rusk observe, "The group recognized that the key to an intuitive structure depends on the organization behind it and the flexibility of the structure to include seamlessly 'not-yet-created' content" (1996). While this precept drove the Web Committee, it was difficult for the content work group to accept it with enough confidence to actually expend the necessary energy to develop new content without knowing that it would have a definite home on the new website. If the content work group had been able to internalize this concept, it would have been much easier to have the visual design work group separated from the content group and have both groups be equally productive. The content work group collected system-wide library forms and policies that needed to be posted on the new site, revised and updated information currently on the site, and verified information once it had been posted on the test site developed by library systems.

Subject Access to Electronic Resources Work Group. The subject access to electronic resources work group had the most clearly defined mission–to provide subject access to University Libraries' electronic resources. In the former website, the electronic resources were presented in two alphabetical lists, one list for databases and one list for electronic journals. However, as the number of electronic resources available continued to grow, this method of access was no longer as viable as it had been. Many of the specialized databases were lost in long alphabetical listings and the patrons who would benefit most from these databases were not necessarily finding them.

LORA, Library Online Resource Access, is a result of the work of the subject access work group. LORA is the dynamic, database-driven interface that now provides access to the library's electronic resources. Many issues had to be resolved during the development phases of LORA. Often work group members met with public services librarians throughout the library system for feedback because of the implications it would have on how they performed their duties. Some of the questions that needed to be answered were the following:

- Should the new system have a new identity and name or should it continue as ejournals and databases?
- Should "free" web resources as well as paid resource subscriptions be included in the system?
- What subject areas will be listed? Should the subjects be broad, for example, humanities, social sciences, life sciences, physical sciences, etc., or should the subjects be more specific such as Library of Congress subject headings?
- Should select resources that are held locally be included like databases available on CD-ROM rather than via the Internet or should we limit the system to only those items that can be accessible from the Internet?

The work group recommended that the system be named since it was a new reference service. The new service needed a name to brand it with existing library resources. It was also decided that free resources such as Internet links and search engines would be included as would locally held resources like CD-ROMs and print indexes. The work group utilized a list of subjects based on degree-granting disciplines at the university since librarians already had assigned liaison responsibilities for those subject areas and could assume responsibility for updating those subject areas within the system.

After the launch of the new website in January 2002, the Web Committee continued to exist with the same membership. This allowed the committee to reflect on what had been done and have time to make needed improvements. The same work groups of the previous semester, however, were no longer needed so new work groups were formed to better reflect the tasks that still needed to be done. A quality control work group thoroughly scrutinized the new website for inconsistencies and misinformation. Once problems were identified, the Electronic Services Coordinator compiled a prioritized list of needed changes for systems from which they worked. The intranet work group was established to provide a framework for development for the second phase of the website–the library personnel intranet. The visual design work group was charged with revisiting the design from last semester and making improvements. After receiving feedback from users who were frustrated because there was only a picture of the main library on the site's front page rather than content, a new front page was proposed that would have more information on it yet maintain some of the needed white space. New colors were also suggested for the navigation bars that were compliant with the suggested web colors published by the University.

THE ROLE OF THE ELECTRONIC SERVICES COORDINATOR

Shortly before the first meeting of the newly formed Web Committee, University Libraries hired its first Electronic Services Coordinator (ESC). This position was created with a half-time appointment to the library's reference department and a half-time appointment reporting directly to the Director of Public Services. One of the primary functions of this position was to act as a liaison between the public services personnel and the library systems office. The person in this position was appointed as a member of the library Web Committee and played a key role in keeping channels of communication open between library personnel both on and off of the Web Committee. Fowler discusses the role of coordinators in this capacity and explains that one of the biggest challenges faced by someone filling this role is to "know the languages and concerns of both corners, and to be reasonably fluent enough in both of them so as to be able to relate to each other's concerns in terms that they can both understand" (2000). Since the ESC was new to the profession and to her position, she was learning both languages simultaneously and had to rely heavily on her colleagues for patience and training.

The ESC was a recent MLIS (Master in Library and Information Studies) graduate and had spent several years working throughout the library in various student and classified staff positions. The ESC had established working relationships with library personnel and had worked directly with those serving on the Web Committee in their various departments. This gave the ESC unique insight into some of the demands and needs of various departments on the library website as well as how it was utilized. The ESC communicated and negotiated with both the public services areas and systems office personnel. The ESC developed a monitoring process on who should be doing what and gathered the necessary content for the new website from the appropriate library personnel. It was beneficial for the Web Committee to have a designated member who was responsible for keeping lines of communication open, who could test new ideas with library personnel, and who could communicate necessary feedback information to the interested parties. Since this was a newly created position, the ESC was able to build in time for web development and communicating changes with personnel from the beginning rather than having to try to work it into an already full workload or to cutback on existing responsibilities.

THE ROLE OF SYSTEMS

The library systems office played an integral role in the development of the new website. While the public and technical services personnel were responsible for developing content and suggesting layout and design for the new website, the library systems office was responsible for actually creating the new site. The systems staff was heavily represented on the Web Committee and had a representative in every work group. This ensured that work groups did not spend hours developing ideas that were unreasonable from a technical standpoint and helped groups get immediate feedback and suggestions from the systems office. In addition, public and technical services personnel could be informed of the technological limitations faced by the systems office and some of the difficulties experienced by off-campus users.

At the outset, one important separation of duties was made that greatly impacted systems mode of operation–public and technical services personnel would provide the web content, and the systems personnel would provide the technical expertise to make content available.

One of the goals of the website redesign was to move to a database-driven web environment and away from the thousands of individually designed HTML pages. As Adalian and Swanson note about managing static HTML pages, "A manageable collection of current static documents quickly became an unmanageable collection of static documents containing outdated information" (2001). Moving to a database-driven website allowed public and technical services personnel to focus on developing content for the new site rather than working on improving their HTML skills. In addition, in a database-driven environment, updating procedures are expedited because changes are only made in one place and all of the pages that utilize that piece of information reflect that change. This meant that systems spent a good deal of time developing interfaces on the staff intranet that would enable public and technical services personnel the ability to control the content within the database but would not compromise the unified look of the website.

MARKETING THE WEBSITE

Before the new University Libraries website could launch in January 2002, it was essential that library faculty, staff and students have the opportunity to preview the new website and make suggestions. The first marketing task was to promote the new website internally. Two meetings were held in late November to provide an opportunity for feedback from all library faculty and staff about the work of the Web Committee. The new website structure was presented and the attendees had the opportunity to ask questions and make suggestions. An evaluation form was developed to solicit feedback from the participants after the web preview sessions.

The website preview sessions provided valuable information for the Web Committee to consider including suggestions about the font selected, the naming of LORA, and inconsistent use of terminology. Attendees liked the increased ease of navigation throughout the website as well as subject access to electronic resources. The committee was also asked to consider some new sections such as information for visitors and for new students as well as providing a printer-friendly version of the website.

In addition to marketing the website internally, marketing the new website to the campus community was also important to the Web Committee and the library. Traditional means were utilized, such as press releases to the campus newspaper and faculty newsletter. Bookmarks were developed, and an announcement was posted on the current website. The reference librarians shared the information with the faculty liaisons in the various departments. All library public service faculty, staff, and students were asked to verbally present the information to patrons when and where possible. Librarians also discussed the change in the website during their library instruction classes. In addition, an e-mail was distributed to library liaisons and department chairs about the transition to the new website. The Director of Public Services and the Systems Director gave presentations for the student government leaders, the University Libraries Committee, and the University Libraries Student Advisory Committee about the features of the new website.

Transition to the new University Libraries website was made during winter intersession in order to minimize impact on the campus community. A briefing session about how to introduce the new website to students and faculty was organized by the Web Committee chair and the Electronic Services Coordinator. Eight sessions were organized on "Navigating the Library Website" for the campus community in late January and early February. A one page fact sheet introducing LORA (Library Online Resource Access) was created to supplement these sessions.

After the new website was introduced in early January 2002, the committee sought feedback from the campus community. Library faculty talked about the change in their library instruction classes and asked the students for feedback. The subject librarians also asked their library liaisons for feedback during individual reference transactions. The librarians often illustrated that the website had an electronic feedback form developed by the Web Committee that enabled users to provide anonymous feedback about the new website. This opened channels of communication that were not present in the previous version of the site.

IMPROVING REFERENCE SERVICES THROUGH REDESIGN OF THE WEBSITE

The new website improved reference services to the libraries' patrons in many ways. One of the most obvious improvements was the addition of LORA (Library Online Resource Access) which provided subject access to the University Libraries electronic resources. This elevated some of the more specialized subject databases that had gotten lost in the long, alphabetical lists of databases and ejournals and made patrons aware that such tools existed. LORA also provided subject librarians a unified avenue for presenting patrons with select Internet links, specialized indexes, and CD-ROMs. With the previous website, librarians who knew HTML or how to use web-publishing software could create web-based subject guides that provided this same information, but not all librarians felt comfortable with this medium so some subject areas were lacking these guides. The interface developed by Systems enabled all subject librarians to create and update these lists of resources for their subject areas with minimal technical knowledge required. Since Systems controlled presentation while librarians controlled content, all subject areas had the same presentation regardless of the resources listed. This improved services for users conducting interdisciplinary research; once they familiarized themselves with the LORA interface, they could expect the same types of materials for all subject areas they may want to investigate.

The new navigation bar and consistent design throughout the website made the new site more intuitive than the previous site had been. Users see the same navigation bars on every page within the site and they can expect to see the same types of information for each area within the site. Each unit within the library has its personnel roster, contact information, and a brief description of what the unit does within the library system posted on its page. This enables users to make educated choices about which unit they need to contact for their needs and makes the contact information readily available. Listing branch libraries and special collections on the side navigation bar increased their visibility and potentially alerted patrons that such collections existed. In addition to this, the library catalog, LORA, electronic reserve, e-mail a librarian, and other heavily utilized services are available from every page within the site so patrons can easily find them regardless of how deeply they roam within the site.

One of the more underlying improvements to our reference service is a result of moving to a database-driven website. Content is more easily and uniformly updated because one change in the database is reflected throughout the site wherever that information is displayed. Patrons can easily find the most current information and there is no conflicting information on the website. With the previous website, a circulation policy change may result in having to update six unique, static pages each maintained by a different person within University Libraries. There was typically a significant time lag between when the policy changed and when that change was accurately reflected throughout the entire website. Patrons often got misinformation or conflicting information from the previous library website; however, with the new site, this is not the case. In addition, changes can be made more rapidly to the site because those responsible for the policy changes often have the appropriate permissions to make changes on the website shortly after the policy change has been implemented. By design, decision-makers are no longer reliant on systems to make content changes on the website.

EVOLUTION OF THE WEB COMMITTEE

Before the Web Committee concluded its year, the members discussed a new Web Committee structure to meet the continuing need to update and refine the library website. Rather than a research and development model, a new Web Committee structure is needed for improved communication between the various library departments and branches. A web steering committee comprised of the Director of Public Services, Director of Systems, and the Electronic Services Coordinator is the leadership group for the new web liaison committee. As Guenther points out, "Without a strong governance structure and process in place, Web development priorities are based on a strategy of 'who yells the loudest,' not necessarily on which priorities have the greatest strategic impact for the organization" (2001). The web steering committee prioritizes suggested web improvements and takes into consideration other demands on systems and public services personnel.

In the Web Committee there were representatives from a cross-section of public services, technical services and systems personnel; however, not every branch and department was represented equitably. In the Web Liaison Committee, each branch and department provides one representative to the Web Liaison Committee which will meet more infrequently than the previous Web Committee. As Davidson and Rusk discuss about their experiences with creating websites using teams, after the site has been launched, there must be continuous thought about maintaining the site and making improvements as necessary (1996). The primary purpose of the web liaison committee is to provide an active channel of two-way communication between the library staff and the web steering committee. The new content that has been added since the Web Liaison Committee has been active includes an online tutorial for library instruction, a virtual tour of the main library, branches and collections, and a further expansion of the staff intranet.

EVALUATION OF THE WEBSITE
AND OF THE COLLABORATIVE PROCESS

During the summer of 2001 the chair of the Web Committee attended several sessions of a course offered by the School of Library and Information Studies. One of the elements of the course, "Design and Implementation of Networked Information Services," was to evaluate library websites with a standard web evaluation tool. The students in the course offered University Libraries a critique of their website that included site planning and design, navigation, page design, and page layout. The students included a written evaluation that was shared with the Web Committee during the fall of 2001. During the summer of 2002, the same course was offered, and a new group of students evaluated the new University Libraries website that had been launched in January. The students' remarks about the new website were consistently positive about their ability to navigate through the site to find the reference services needed. In particular, the students cited improved access to electronic resources by subject as well as consistent presentation of the information, the ability to return to the library home page from any location within the website as well as questioning the use of a large graphic on the front page rather than more content.

The website feedback forms identified a wide range of user issues that included browser compatibility, shift of content to secondary levels, lack of understanding terminology as well as favorable comments about increased white space, improved navigation, subject access and consistent style throughout the website. User feedback was particularly critical from off-campus users because they brought to the Web Committee's attention problems that were not present for on-campus users. Through feedback forms and telephone calls, some users indicated that they thought the library had cancelled all subscriptions to databases and electronic journals because there was no longer a link labeled either databases or ejournals directly on the front page of the library website. Usage statistics reported by Systems, however, indicated that the use of LORA was significantly increased over the lists of ejournals and databases lists that previously existed. In the first quarter of 2001, the usage of the ejournals and databases lists accounted for 22% of the total library website activity. During the first quarter of 2002, usage of LORA accounted for 33% of the total website activity.

At the final meeting of the Web Committee meeting, the chair asked the members of the committee to evaluate the group process, the final product, and the enhanced services available through the new website.

Challenges faced by the members of the Web Committee included the following:

- learning to be flexible and compromise;
- accepting that a voice is not a vote in a collaborative environment;
- breaking into work groups to produce results;
- preparing for an increase in projected time for new projects;
- recognizing the necessity of continued patience over time;
- relinquishing control over web pages; and,
- understanding the implications of moving to a database-driven web environment.

The chair of the committee felt that the research and development mission of the Web Committee was important to the visibility of the library website to the library staff. The time table was ambitious.

CONCLUSION

Developing a collaborative culture was a major time investment for every member of the Web Committee. Cooperative learning, communicating, and forming an environment where testing and making mistakes was allowed helped to build a foundation for the Web Committee that was essential to the learning process of the group. Not every objective was met with the newly updated website; however, the major objectives were accomplished within a well-publicized set of strategies that helped transform reluctance to change into confidence and focused energy.

Building reference services that meet the needs of today's students and faculty requires continuous testing, feedback, analysis, and development. What does it take to build enduring reference services through the library website? Committee members asked themselves this one basic question many times throughout the year. The answer is simple: focus on users' needs, design a website to meet these needs, and be open to suggestions for improvement. The purpose of the Web Committee was not simply to take the web structure that had previously existed and repackage it but rather to examine the way in which students and faculty use the library website. The Web Committee's research and development focus combined with a collaborative environment provided a positive impetus for change to the library website and improved reference services to the university community.

REFERENCES

Adalian, Paul T. and Judy Swanson (2001), "Locally Developed Web-Enabled Databases: New Roles and Opportunities," *Reference Services Review* 29 (3), 238-252.

Bunker, Geri and Greg Zick (1999), "Collaboration as a Key to Digital Library Development," *D-Lib Magazine* 5 (3). Available at http://www.dlib.org/dlib/march99/bunker/03bunker.html.

Davidson, Jeanne and Cherie Rusk (1996), "Creating a University Web in a Team Environment," *Journal of Academic Librarianship* 22 (July), 302-305.

Dupuis, John and Patti Ryan (2002) "Bridging the Two Cultures: A Collaborative Approach to Managing Electronic Resources," *Issues in Science and Technology Librarianship* (Spring). Available at http://www.istl.org/02-spring/article1.html.

Fowler, David C. (2000), "Information Technology and Collection Development Departments in the Academic Library: Striving to Reach a Common Understanding," *Collection Management* 25 (1-2), 17-36.

Guenther, Kim (2001), "Web Site Management: Effective Web Governance Structures," *Online* 25 (2), 70-72.

Jagodzinski, Cecile, Jim Cunningham, Pam Day, Sharon Naylor, and Elizabeth Schobernd (1997), "Cooperative Web Weaving: The Team Approach to Web Site Development at Illinois State University," *Journal of Interlibrary Loan, Document Delivery & Information Supply* 8 (2), 1-20.

Manning, Jamie (2002), "Creating the Customer-Obsessed Web Team," *EContent* 25 (1), 37-40.

McMullen, Susan (2001), "Usability Testing in a Library Web Site Redesign Project," *Reference Services Review* 29 (1), 7-22.

Soete, George J., comp. (1998), *Use of Teams in ARL Libraries*. Washington, DC: Association of Research Libraries.

Smith, Susan, Rosalind Tedford, and Giz Womack (2001). "Make it a Team Effort." *NetConnect* (Winter), 18-20.

Stover, Mark (1997), "Library Web Sites: Mission and Function in the Networked Organization," *Computers in Libraries* 17 (November/December), 55-57.

The Role of Cooperation
in Creating a Library Online Tutorial

Eve M. Diel

Theresa K. Flett

SUMMARY. Reference librarians at St. Charles Community College discovered the benefits of cooperation when they began the process of creating an online library tutorial. In the fall of 1999, librarians realized that their walk-in library sessions were becoming ineffective due to poor attendance by students. The tours didn't fit into on-campus students' busy schedules, and failed to serve distance students at all. Two reference librarians decided to work together to create a web-based tutorial introducing students to library online resources. It was an informal process that started with information gathering on what tutorials exist, how they were developed and what type of software was used. After the librarians decided on the format and appropriate software, they brought together their creative and technical strengths to design an appealing and functional tutorial. To create a "virtual tour" of the library's physical layout, the librarians also collaborated with the Instructional Support Center, a group of educational technology specialists who are part of SCC's community college consortium. The tutorial was completed in only a

Eve M. Diel is Librarian, Parkway West High School, 14653 Clayton Road, Ballwin, MO 63001 (E-mail: ediel@pkwy.k12.mo.us). At the time this was written, she was Reference Librarian, St. Charles Community College, St. Peters, MO. Theresa K. Flett is Reference Librarian, St. Charles Community College, 4601 Mid Rivers Mall Drive, St. Peters, MO 63376 (E-mail: tflett@stchas.edu).

[Haworth co-indexing entry note]: "The Role of Cooperation in Creating a Library Online Tutorial." Diel, Eve M., and Theresa K. Flett. Co-published simultaneously in *The Reference Librarian* (The Haworth Information Press, an imprint of The Haworth Press, Inc.) No. 83/84, 2003, pp. 175-182; and: *Cooperative Reference: Social Interaction in the Workplace* (ed: Celia Hales Mabry) The Haworth Information Press, an imprint of The Haworth Press, Inc., 2003, pp. 175-182. Single or multiple copies of this article are available for a fee from The Haworth Document Delivery Service [1-800-HAWORTH, 9:00 a.m. - 5:00 p.m. (EST). E-mail address: docdelivery@haworthpress.com].

year, partly because working in a small library allows for constant contact between the librarians, but also due to the efficiency of using cooperation. This successful collaborative project eventually won the Missouri Community College Association's 2001 Technology Innovation Award. *[Article copies available for a fee from The Haworth Document Delivery Service: 1-800-HAWORTH. E-mail address: <docdelivery@haworthpress.com> Website: <http://www.HaworthPress.com> © 2003 by The Haworth Press, Inc. All rights reserved.]*

KEYWORDS. Online tutorials, librarian collaboration, online library instruction, web-based instruction

Creating an online tutorial is an effort requiring collaboration and cooperation. The creation of an online tutorial seems almost mandatory in academic libraries today, given the number of articles written, presentations given, and listserv discussions on the topic. The technology and feasibility of the project are often stressed in these discussions, and it is important that these issues are discussed. The interpersonal cooperation, however, that is vital in making such a project successful is often not mentioned at all. As Lippincott notes in her article "Working Together," no matter how much each party working on a project knows about technology or content, the project will not be a successful collaboration unless the partners have mutual goals for the project (Lippincott, 1998). Luckily, at our college, both of us worked together to develop common goals for the project and also enjoyed working together. Each librarian brought her own strengths and ideas to the project. We also learned a great deal from each other by the project's completion, making the project a learning experience for us as well as its users.

When looking at other online tutorial projects, many similarities appear. In most cases, libraries decided to create a tutorial for a few major reasons: to free up librarian time, to provide alternatives to the traditional orientation to the library, to eliminate underutilized walk-in tours, and to accommodate different learning styles (Ardis, 1998; Tricarico, 2001). Many articles on how to design tutorials discuss the importance of interactivity and developing clear goals for the tutorial (Dewald, 1999b). Most articles written emphasize the fact that these tutorials cannot replace the effectiveness of in-person instruction but can enhance traditional instruction (Dewald, 1999a). In our case we were also hoping to free up time to provide more specialized instruction to classes at their time of need.

Some differences arise in the process of the design and scope of the tutorials. Some libraries have a large budget with many resources. Many have a few dedicated individuals making do with what they can get their hands on or what help is available to them (Gray, 1999). Some of the plans are very organized with a detailed work plan and organization of labor (Ardis, 1998). Many of the plans depend on the expertise of other departments, or, in our case, consortium resources. At SCC, we have a small library with two busy reference librarians who decided to work on the project. Due to our library's size, we have many professional responsibilities and the time to work on such an intense project is limited. Such a project is clearly impossible for one librarian to take on alone. Both of us have a strong understanding of web page creation and design, but because we wear so many hats in our small library, neither of us has the time to become web technology experts. Because of our limited time and resources, we had to work closely together to create the best tutorial we could with our own knowledge and abilities, and to take advantage of technological expertise and software available to us through our college consortium. As one article notes, "a lack of resources or time or both has often led independent groups to join forces to accomplish goals, and so to collaborate" (Broms, 2001). This idea is very true in a small library, and our collaboration with each other and our college consortium grew directly from this lack.

The collaborative development of the tutorial began in late 1999 when the SCC reference librarians attended various library conference sessions discussing the use of online tutorials. One of the issues mentioned in the sessions was the difficulty in designing a tutorial that was truly interactive–in other words, requiring the students to interact with the computer more than simply clicking an arrow to move to the next screen. We also read several listserv discussions about library tutorials. Since we had been having problems with scheduling our walk-in tours to be convenient to students, and since the distance students could not attend these sessions at all, we decided that creating a tutorial would be an excellent alternative.

We began by developing objectives to be met by the tutorial. We wanted to be certain that our tutorial covered all the information given in the walk-in sessions, including the physical tour of the library. We also wanted to be certain the tutorial was truly interactive. We felt that it was very important to include some type of assessment module, letting us know how the students were performing on the tutorial, and helping us identify areas to improve. We wanted to include a survey component to get feedback from the students on the strengths and weaknesses of the tutorial, so we could make further improvements.

Before we started on the project, we wanted to be certain to communicate with our faculty about the project to determine their reaction and level of support. We sent a memo to the faculty to inform them of the possibility of creating an online library tutorial. We followed up this memo with a survey to learn whether they would support this type of library instruction. When the survey results were returned with feedback in favor of the tutorial, we began the design process.

With the requirements for our interactive tutorial in mind, we determined the type of technology and software that would enable us to meet them. We knew that we wanted the tutorial to be delivered through the Web, so students could complete the tutorial at any time and at any place with Web access. We realized that we would need some type of course development software to assist us in making quizzes and keeping statistics. We would also need a web design software program to help us create interactive aspects of the tutorial using JavaScript, since our JavaScript knowledge is at a basic level. We wanted to create an interactive imagemap using library floor plans to give students a "virtual tour" of the physical library.

The first step was to determine the course development software to use for the project. St. Charles Community College is involved in the Gateway Community College Consortium which uses WebCT for its online course development software. We discussed our needs with the staff of the Instructional Support Center (ISC), the technology support team of the Gateway consortium. Since WebCT had the quiz, statistics, and survey functions that we needed to meet our objectives, and had the added benefit of being used and supported on our campus, we decided to use WebCT to deliver the course on the Web. The ISC staff also worked with us by providing training on the WebCT course development software and offering suggestions as to how it might best be used to reach our goals.

Another objective to be met was to create some type of interactive floor plan to orient students to the physical library, but we felt that the technical knowledge needed to create this floor plan was beyond our abilities. Again, we turned to the ISC for assistance. When we mentioned the possibility of creating a "virtual tour" of the library, they suggested that members of their staff had the ability to create a 3-D rendering of the library's floor plan. This floor plan could include clickable links on various areas in the library and 360° views of the reference room and the second floor. The reference librarians and the ISC discussed this aspect of the project in great detail and arrived at a design that both parties found useful and feasible. The librarians supplied their content expertise, including a copy of the floor plan and various locations to include, plus the text of the links and explanations of the different areas, while the ISC used their technical expertise to make the content into a visually appealing, interactive floor plan. The end result was a very effective and engaging presentation of the library's layout that pleased the ISC team and us as well.

Our next need was to find web page development software that would help us design visually appealing web pages including interactivity with JavaScript. To identify possible software, we collaborated in a casual way with librarians throughout the country via listserv discussions. We queried several library listservs to learn about the experiences of other librarians in creating online tutorials and the software they found beneficial. From the ensuing discussions, we learned about Dreamweaver web development software to create professional-looking web pages. Dreamweaver has an optional add-on software, called CourseBuilder, which allows the web designer to create JavaScript applications in the form of questions providing immediate feedback after the user chooses an answer. We downloaded a trial copy of Dreamweaver with CourseBuilder and found it very intuitive and easy to use, so we decided to purchase the software to create our web pages for the tutorial.

Our collaborative efforts with various groups allowed us to be very creative and innovative in developing our online tutorial. We started from scratch, so we had full creative license in coming up with graphics and layout allowing us to freely draw from our own knowledge and the knowledge of our collaborators. One of us is very creative with design and layout while the other is quick to learn software applications, so by bringing these strengths together we were able to quickly and efficiently create the content pages on the Web. Because the software was new to both of us, we worked closely with each other as we taught ourselves to use it, sharing any tricks we learned to make the process easier.

Although creating an online tutorial is not unusual for libraries today, there are several features of our tutorial that make it truly unique and innovative. For example, although we used WebCT software, which allows the designer to customize a standard web page menu, we created our own web pages outside of WebCT using Dreamweaver. This allowed us the freedom of creating our tutorial's distinctive look, while still enabling us to utilize the powerful tracking and statistical components of the WebCT software. Many library tutorials do not track their students in this way, but we wanted to gain measurable feedback through quiz and usage statistics as well as student survey feedback to help us maintain and improve the tutorial. Another distinctive feature of our tutorial is the use of web page frames. This technique allows students to access the library catalog and databases through the main web page frame, and to follow instructions from the tutorial in the side frame. This use of frames makes our tutorial truly interactive, because students must interact with the databases and the catalog by typing in search terms, looking at their search results, and selecting items to view in more detail. We also consider the "virtual tour" created with the co-operation of the Instructional Support Center of the Gateway Community College Consortium to be an innovative aspect of our tutorial, setting it apart from other library tutorials.

To maintain communication with faculty about the tutorial after it was completed in the summer of 2000, we sent out a memo and e-mail to all faculty advertising the new tutorial and inviting them to try it. We also presented a session on Information Literacy at the Fall Faculty Inservice and presented our new tutorial to them and again invited them to try it out and to suggest it to their students. To reach the adjunct faculty, we discussed the tutorial at the Adjunct Faculty Inservice and presented information on the tutorial in a handout.

To evaluate the project we used informal feedback from faculty, the amount of students completing the tutorial, students' performance on the quizzes, and comments from the student survey. The feedback from the faculty has been very positive, since their students do not have to wait for a scheduled tour. We have eliminated the poorly attended walk-in sessions and as of August 2002 we have had 1,241 students access the tutorial. The students have performed well on the quizzes, with the average score on the Magazines/Newspaper Indexes quiz at 88.0 out of 100 and the Archway Online Catalog quiz at 88.3 out of 100. The majority of feedback from the student survey has been very positive. Overall, students find the tutorial very helpful in their efforts to find information in the library. Students are pleased that the tutorial is available to them at any time on the Internet and it is something they can do on their own time at home. The SCC reference librarians were also very honored that their tutorial was selected as the recipient of the 2001 Missouri Community College Association's Technology Innovation Award.

The tutorial met our objectives of allowing both on-campus and distance students to have the benefit of library instruction. It allows on-campus students to fit library instruction into their busy schedules, and is accessible to distance students. The web-based tutorial allows students to access the tutorial from any computer with Web access, at any time. The self-paced nature of the online tutorial enables students to take as much time as they need and to repeat sections if necessary. The tutorial is also truly interactive, since students must not only click the arrows to move from page to page, but must also choose answers to short self-tests and search within the databases and the catalog.

The tutorial has had a highly positive impact on reference staff productivity. The walk-in sessions were very time consuming. Each walk-in session took an hour of staff time and was generally only attended by one to five students. Combining the fall and spring semesters, staff devoted approximately 88 hours of time to giving the walk-in tours, and usually a maximum of only 352 students total were in attendance for the semester. With our online tutorial, the only staff time required is a few minutes to answer occasional student questions about logging in or other housekeeping information. For fall 2000-spring 2001, we had 699 students access the online tutorial, and for fall 2001-spring 2002, we had 542 students access the tutorial. The tutorial, therefore, has nearly doubled the amount of students reached per semester, yet cut staff time down to almost nothing. This has dramatically freed up reference librarians' time to do more specialized instruction for specific classes.

Our cooperative project was a definite success because it met all our objectives and had a positive impact on staff productivity. Without the collaboration between the reference librarians themselves, cooperation with the Instructional Support Center, communication with faculty as to our goals and objectives, and casual collaboration with librarians around the country, this successful project could never have taken place.

REFERENCES

Ardis, Susan B. (1998), "Creating Internet-Based Tutorials," *Information Outlook* 2 (October), 17-20.

Broms, Susan K. (2001), "Perspectives on Librarian Collaborations–A Survey of AALL Chapters," *Legal Reference Services Quarterly* 20(3), 65-90.

Dewald, Nancy H. (1999), "Transporting Good Library Instruction Practices into the Web Environment: An Analysis of Online Tutorials," *Journal of Academic Librarianship* 25 (January), 26-32.

Dewald, Nancy H. (1999), "Web-Based Library Instruction: What is Good Pedagogy?" *Information Technology & Libraries* 18 (March), 26-31.

Gray, David (1999), "Online at Your Own Pace: Web-Based Tutorials in Community College Libraries," *Virginia Libraries* 45 (January-March), 9-10.

Lippincott, Joan K. (1998), "Working Together: Building Collaboration Between Libraries and Information Technologists," *Information Technology & Libraries* 17 (June), 83-84+. Retrieved May 16, 2002, from First Search Periodical Abstracts database.

Tricarico, Mary A., von Daum Tholl, Susan, & O'Malley, Elena (2001), "Interactive Online Instruction for Library Research: The Small Academic Library Experience," *Journal of Academic Librarianship* 27 (May), 220-223.

E-Mail Reference:
Improving Service
by Working Cooperatively

Sharon Ladenson

SUMMARY. E-mail reference service provides complex challenges, but the service can be planned effectively and improved through cooperative work among reference staff and various library departments. Staff members from the Michigan State University Libraries have engaged in extensive cooperative work to evaluate, improve, and maintain effective e-mail reference services. Two library committees and an e-mail reference team have developed new service procedures, and have worked with other library departments to improve e-mail reference service. This article explores the collaborative work of the MSU committees, and discusses how e-mail reference has improved through cooperative work. *[Article copies available for a fee from The Haworth Document Delivery Service: 1-800-HAWORTH. E-mail address: <docdelivery@haworthpress.com> Website: <http://www.HaworthPress.com> © 2003 by The Haworth Press, Inc. All rights reserved.]*

KEYWORDS. Academic libraries, collaboration, cooperation, electronic reference, e-mail, library committees, virtual reference

Sharon Ladenson is Communications Bibliographer and Reference Librarian, Michigan State University, 100 Main Library, East Lansing, MI 48824-1048 (E-mail: ladenson@msu.edu).

[Haworth co-indexing entry note]: "E-Mail Reference: Improving Service by Working Cooperatively." Ladenson, Sharon. Co-published simultaneously in *The Reference Librarian* (The Haworth Information Press, an imprint of The Haworth Press, Inc.) No. 83/84, 2003, pp. 183-191; and: *Cooperative Reference: Social Interaction in the Workplace* (ed: Celia Hales Mabry) The Haworth Information Press, an imprint of The Haworth Press, Inc., 2003, pp. 183-191. Single or multiple copies of this article are available for a fee from The Haworth Document Delivery Service [1-800-HAWORTH, 9:00 a.m. - 5:00 p.m. (EST). E-mail address: docdelivery@haworthpress.com].

183

How can collaborative work enhance and improve e-mail reference service? The literature on e-mail reference indicates that the service provides unique challenges, and can be planned effectively and improved through collaborative work. Members of Michigan State University (MSU) library committees were recently charged with the task of evaluating and improving e-mail reference service, and have made collective decisions that changed service procedures. This article provides an overview of the collaborative efforts and accomplishments of the MSU committees, and illustrates how e-mail reference service has improved through cooperative work.

The literature on e-mail reference provides evidence that the service is complex, and differs greatly from in-person and telephone reference. Nonverbal communication (such as facial expression and tone of voice) can facilitate reference interviews in-person and on the telephone, and e-mail reference lacks such communication (Garnsey and Powell, 2000). The lack of real-time interaction in e-mail reference can effect significant delays in answering questions; e-mail reference interviews can last for days or weeks (Abels, 1996). Consequently, staff who do e-mail reference might search for information before the reference interview has been completed, or skip the negotiation process altogether (Abels, 1996). Some librarians indicate that they prefer to quickly provide an answer, rather than respond with additional questions; sometimes, a message containing several possible answers is provided in response to a single question (Lederer, 2001).

As a complex and difficult task, e-mail reference requires cooperative work among various library departments. Bibliographers can contribute by answering specialized reference questions in their subject areas (Garnsey and Powell, 2000). On the other hand, e-mail reference staff may need to refer service questions to other departments, such as Circulation or Interlibrary Loan. Librarians from the State University of New York (SUNY) at Buffalo analyzed 485 e-mail reference questions, and discovered that 30% of the questions " . . . were book renewal requests, questions regarding borrowing privileges, and requests to have books held at the circulation desk" (Bushallow-Wilbur, DeVinney, and Whitcomb, 1996).

Cooperative work can also facilitate effective planning of e-mail reference services. Weissman (2001) recommends that staff should be consulted when making fundamental decisions about e-mail reference policy and procedures. Furthermore, O'Neill (1999) asserts that working closely with staff when planning e-mail reference service can help "overcome initial resistance" to providing the service.

Members of the library staff from Michigan State University (MSU) have worked cooperatively to plan and improve e-mail reference service. Staff members have worked together on committees to evaluate the library's e-mail reference service, recommend changes for service procedures, and begin implementing such changes. During the summer of 2000, the MSU Libraries' Head of Reference organized numerous meetings for librarians to discuss issues regarding e-mail reference service. In the fall of 2000, an Electronic Reference Services Committee, comprised of four librarians, was developed to complete several tasks, including (among others) reviewing the discussions that took place during the summer, and recommending changes to improve e-mail reference services. After reviewing the minutes of the reference meetings conducted during the summer of 2000, the Electronic Reference Services Committee determined that MSU librarians' biggest concern about electronic reference was the difficulty in conducting a reference interview by e-mail (Jones, Schaubman, Wells, and Young, 2001).

The MSU Libraries' Electronic Reference Services Committee made several recommendations regarding e-mail reference service. Committee members suggested revising the MSU Libraries' web pages designed for submitting e-mail reference questions, in order to facilitate and improve the process of expressing reference questions electronically (Jones et al., 2001). The committee also recommended developing standard methods and procedures for handling referrals of e-mail questions, identifying e-mail questions that could be answered effectively using canned responses, and, publicizing and promoting e-mail reference in order to increase usage of the service (Jones et al., 2001).

In the fall of 2000, The MSU Libraries' Electronic Reference Services Committee started the process of working collaboratively to recommend and develop new policies and procedures for e-mail reference. During the following year, a larger E-mail Reference Committee was formed to address some of the recommendations of the Electronic Reference Services Committee, and investigate other ways to improve e-mail reference services. The new committee was comprised of four librarians from the Main Library Reference department, one branch librarian, one library assistant, and one staff member from the Systems department. The E-mail Reference Committee developed criteria for evaluating software products for e-mail reference, and identified potential products to review. Committee members also reviewed the MSU Libraries' e-mail reference web pages, and suggested potential changes. In addition, the committee reviewed nearly 700 e-mail reference questions and replies from January 1997 to June 2001, in order to identify questions that could be answered effectively using canned responses. After an initial meeting, members decided to divide the group into three smaller subcommittees to complete the tasks of identifying software products, reviewing the web form, and reading past e-mail reference questions and replies (Bryant, Cooper, Fox, Lorenzen, Volkening, Wells, and Wilson, 2001).

The entire committee worked to develop criteria for selecting software. These criteria included, among others, that software products should be affordable and easy to use, and should allow staff to access and respond to e-mail questions from various locations. The product should also support a database of canned replies, and have the capacity to generate statistical reports. After the committee collectively established the criteria for evaluating products, two subcommittee members identified software programs for the group to review. After examining available products, the committee decided that the programs reviewed did not suit the needs of library. Some products were designed for help desks at private companies rather than for libraries, and, consequently, committee members discovered that such programs were poorly suited for e-mail reference. Other products were eliminated because the MSU Libraries did not have the technological resources to support them. Consequently, the subcommittee recommended that the library should consider designing its own product to use for e-mail reference, since the products currently available did not meet the needs of the library (Bryant et al., 2001).

The committee also worked collectively to determine necessary features for the web pages used to submit e-mail reference questions. Committee members decided that the pages should include a brief description of the nature and scope of the service, and provide links to alternative sources for answers, such as web research guides created by MSU Librarians. The committee also recommended adding a privacy statement, and, consequently, the e-mail web page subcommittee worked to draft a privacy statement to include on the e-mail reference home page (Bryant et al., 2001).

Reviewing the MSU Libraries' e-mail web pages also prompted the committee to assess and recommend a change regarding a specific service policy. In the past, the e-mail reference web pages indicated that the service was only for users affiliated with Michigan State University. Committee members pointed out that the library provides reference service to nonuniversity patrons over the phone and in-person, and that the policy should remain consistent for e-mail reference. Consequently, the committee also recommended eliminating the statement indicating that e-mail reference was limited to patrons affiliated with Michigan State University (Bryant et al., 2001).

Another subcommittee reviewed and categorized nearly 700 e-mail reference questions and replies from January 1997 to June 2001. The subcommittee found that most patrons requested information regarding a specific library collection or service, an index or journal, research strategies, using the library catalog, and ready reference quick facts. In addition, patrons most frequently requested information in the subject areas of biology, business, education, government, history, literature, sociology and psychology. Based on the findings of the subcommittee, the entire E-mail Reference Committee decided that creating canned responses to e-mail reference questions in popular subject areas would improve the quality of responses, and make the service more efficient (Bryant et al., 2001).

The E-mail Reference Committee also made recommendations regarding general procedures and policies. While e-mail reference had been the responsibility of all reference desk staff, the committee recommended that e-mail questions be handled by a smaller group of interested volunteers. E-mail reference volunteers should have the option of answering e-mail reference questions from their offices, or from a reference desk computer used specifically for electronic reference. When answering e-mail questions, staff should initial their responses, in order to provide for efficient handling of follow-up questions and referrals. The committee also recommended developing a formal procedure for following up on referrals, such as requesting that the librarian who makes a referral be notified when the question is answered (Bryant et al., 2001).

In December of 2001, following the e-mail committee's recommendations, the Head of Main Library Reference recruited twelve interested volunteers from the Reference department to participate on an e-mail reference team. The new e-mail team collectively determined routine procedures and guidelines for hours of service and scheduling. Each day of the week, a different team member would be assigned to answer e-mail reference questions. The service would be offered Monday through Friday; questions submitted on the weekends would be answered the following Monday. Librarians assigned to weekday shifts would be responsible for answering questions submitted throughout the day, and the previous evening. For example, a librarian assigned to work a Tuesday shift would be responsible for answering questions submitted from 5:00 p.m. on Monday evening through 5:00 p.m. on Tuesday evening. Librarians assigned to weekend shifts would be responsible for answering questions submitted from 5:00 p.m. on Friday evening through 5:00 p.m. on Sunday evening; such questions would be answered the following Monday. Responses to questions are provided within two business days (Fox and Sowards, 2002).

Since the 2001 E-mail Reference Committee could not find a suitable product for e-mail reference, the current team decided to use the library's Outlook e-mail program to manage e-mail reference questions. Folders were created within the Reference department's e-mail inbox for the purpose of filing e-mail reference questions on a daily basis. For example, if a librarian is assigned to answer e-mail reference questions on a Tuesday, any unanswered question submitted that day would need to be placed in the "Tuesday" folder, where it remains until it is answered. The e-mail team worked with the MSU Libraries' Systems department to allow for team members to access the Reference department's inbox from their office computers.

The 2001 E-mail Reference Committee also recommended using a software product to track data on the numbers and types of questions asked, and provide a database of canned responses. Since a suitable product was not available, one of the current e-mail team members designed a page for the MSU Libraries' Intranet site to facilitate the task of answering and tracking data on e-mail questions. The page provides an electronic form for staff to complete after answering questions; staff members are asked to provide information on the subjects of questions, the print and electronic resources used to respond, and the length of time spent answering each question. Staff also record referrals made to other library departments or sources outside the library, and record questions that have been referred to the Main Library Reference unit.

The Intranet page also includes links to various canned responses created by members of the current team. The e-mail team decided that all responses to questions should include standard opening and closing remarks, and, consequently, canned responses have been developed accordingly, and linked from the Intranet page. E-mail team members also started creating canned replies for basic questions, such as how to use the library catalog to find materials.

Librarians also recognized the necessity of creating and using canned responses to make appropriate referrals. The Reference department, for example, has received a sizeable number of questions regarding circulation and interlibrary loan policies and procedures. Consequently, e-mail reference staff worked cooperatively with staff from the Circulation and Interlibrary Loan departments to create appropriate canned responses for referring patrons to those units. The text of the canned response assures the patron that the question has already been referred to the appropriate department:

> Thank you for using the e-mail reference service of the Michigan State University Libraries.
>
> Your question involves an Interlibrary Loan procedure. In order to provide you with the most complete and current information possible, a copy of this response (including the text of the original question) is being copied to the e-mail account of the Document Delivery/InterLibrary Loan unit of the MSU Libraries: ill@mail.lib.msu.edu. You can expect a more detailed reply from them within the next two business days.
>
> In the meantime, you may be able to answer some aspect of your question by browsing Web pages created by the Document Delivery/Interlibrary Loan unit, at http://www.lib.msu.edu/docd/.
>
> We hope this referral will yield the information you need. Please feel free to contact us again.
>
> Main Library Reference
> Michigan State University Libraries. (Forro and Sowards, 2002)

Following the recommendations made by the previous committees, the e-mail team revised the e-mail reference home page. The newly revised page provides a brief description of the service, and includes selected links to reference resources, bibliographies and pathfinders designed by MSU Librarians, and web pages of other library departments, such as Circulation, Interlibrary Loan, and Library Distance Learning Services. The old e-mail reference home page provided a link to a form for patrons to submit reference questions, a form that has been condensed, in order to facilitate the process of sending e-mail reference questions. The team also decided to merge the form and the e-mail reference home page, which also facilitates submission of e-mail questions. Since the U.S.A. PATRIOT Act was passed, the e-mail team has recognized the need for a new privacy statement for the e-mail home page; this will require cooperative work with the library administration to ensure that the privacy policy is consistent with the policies of Michigan State University.

E-mail reference service has improved significantly as a result of the cooperative work of the three e-mail reference committees. The new e-mail reference schedule allows librarians to work on questions more thoroughly. Librarians are encouraged to spend time conducting reference interviews over e-mail, rather than answering e-mail questions as quickly as possible during their in-person reference desk shifts. Since the new e-mail team is now comprised of a group of interested volunteers, participants devote considerable time to answering questions thoroughly.

The collaborative work across library departments has provided benefits to the current e-mail reference team. Thanks to the assistance of the libraries' Systems department, e-mail team members can access the Reference department's e-mail inbox from their office computers. This makes the task more convenient, for e-mail reference staff do not have to go to the reference desk several times a day to check the department's inbox for messages. Furthermore, working closely with the staff from Circulation and Interlibrary Loan has improved the process of making referrals to those departments. The new canned responses that have been developed to refer patrons to Circulation and Interlibrary Loan facilitates the referral process.

While e-mail reference provides unique challenges, collaborative work among MSU library staff members has provided for more effective service procedures, and, consequently, the service has improved for patrons and staff. Cooperative work will be required in the future in order to continue to improve and maintain effective e-mail reference service. E-mail team members need to work with bibliographers in order to develop canned responses to questions in specific subject areas. Staff members (including library administrators) need to work together to address issues of privacy in e-mail reference service, particularly since the passage of the U.S.A. PATRIOT Act. Working cooperatively is necessary to provide effective and efficient e-mail reference, and to make the service a manageable task for library staff.

REFERENCES

Abels, E. G. (1996), "The E-Mail Reference Interview," *RQ* 35 (Spring 1996), 345-358.

Bryant, S., Cooper, P., Fox, B., Lorenzen, M., Volkening, T., Wells, A. T., and Wilson T. (2001), *E-Mail Reference Committee Report*. Unpublished report, Michigan State University Libraries.

Bushallow-Wilbur, L., DeVinney, G., and Whitcomb, F. (1996), "Electronic Mail Reference Service: A Study," *RQ* 35 (Spring 1996), 359-371.

Forro, D., and Sowards, S. (2002), *All Interlibrary Loan Related Questions.* Unpublished "canned e-mail reference reply," Michigan State University Libraries.

Fox, B., and Sowards, S. (2002), *E-Mail Reference Procedures.* Unpublished report, Michigan State University Libraries.

Garnsey, B. A. and Powell, R. R. (2000), "Electronic Mail Reference Services in the Public Library," *Reference & User Services Quarterly* 39 (Spring 2000), 245-254.

Jones, R. A., Schaubman, D., Wells, A. T., and Young, C. (2001, January 26), *Report of the MSU Libraries' Electronic Reference Ad Hoc Committee, Fall 2000.* Retrieved November 15, 2002 from http://www.lib.msu.edu/sowards/mlr/electref.html.

Lederer, N. (2001), "E-Mail Reference: Who, When, Where and What Is Asked," *The Reference Librarian* (2001), 55-73.

O'Neill, N. (1999), "E-Mail Reference Service in the Public Library: A Virtual Necessity," *Public Libraries* 38 (Sept./Oct. 1999), 302-303.

Weissman, S. K. (2001), "Considering a Launch?" *Library Journal* 126 (February 1 2001), 49.

Collaboration:
The Key to Unlocking the Dilemma
of Distance Reference Services

Sherry Hawkins Backhus
Terri Pedersen Summey

SUMMARY. Distant education offerings are growing at a phenomenal rate for academic institutions, creating new groups of library users that are remote from the main campus with unique library and research needs. Recent studies examining the needs of this unique and growing population note that reference and research assistance are key services needed. Many institutions have appointed or hired distance education librarians to help provide services to distant learners. They are often, however, one-person operations that function more as coordinators rather than full-service providers. Since the coordinator cannot provide all of the reference services alone, the key to providing these services for distance education students is to create and sustain good working relationships both in the library and with external entities. Offerings to distance students include phone reference and accessibility to online re-

Sherry Hawkins Backhus (E-mail: backhusz@emporia.edu) is Reference Librarian and Instruction Coordinator and Terri Pedersen Summey (E-mail: summeyte@emporia. edu) is Head of Distance Learning Services, Collection Development, and Library Webmaster, both at Emporia State University, W. A. White Library, 1200 Commercial–Box 4051, Emporia, KS 66801.

[Haworth co-indexing entry note]: "Collaboration: The Key to Unlocking the Dilemma of Distance Reference Services." Backhus, Sherry Hawkins, and Terri Pedersen Summey. Co-published simultaneously in *The Reference Librarian* (The Haworth Information Press, an imprint of The Haworth Press, Inc.) No. 83/84, 2003, pp. 193-202; and: *Cooperative Reference: Social Interaction in the Workplace* (ed: Celia Hales Mabry) The Haworth Information Press, an imprint of The Haworth Press, Inc., 2003, pp. 193-202. Single or multiple copies of this article are available for a fee from The Haworth Document Delivery Service [1-800-HAWORTH, 9:00 a.m. - 5:00 p.m. (EST). E-mail address: docdelivery@haworthpress.com].

http://www.haworthpress.com/web/REF
Digital Object Identifier: 10.1300J120v40n83_16

sources, plus virtual reference and often 24/7 services. This article will examine issues and experiences in bringing together different groups to provide reference services to distant learning communities. It will also describe key relationships necessary for keeping distance reference services at an optimal level. *[Article copies available for a fee from The Haworth Document Delivery Service: 1-800-HAWORTH. E-mail address: <docdelivery@haworthpress.com> Website: <http://www.HaworthPress.com> © 2003 by The Haworth Press, Inc. All rights reserved.]*

KEYWORDS. Reference service, distance education, academic libraries, distant education students, virtual reference, distance education librarians, collaboration

Higher education is changing and the way that academic institutions are providing educational opportunities is evolving. Not only are colleges and universities still using traditional means to educate students, they are moving to nontraditional methods. Distance education offerings are growing at a phenomenal rate. This creates both challenges and opportunities for academic libraries.

Challenges include providing services to learning communities remote from the main campus. These groups have unique learning and research needs that libraries struggle to meet with resources and services. Opportunities abound in the ability to design services to meet these needs.

Another challenge is determining the expected current and future services. According to the Association of College and Research Libraries (ACRL) *Guidelines for Distance Learning Library Services* library resources and services must meet the needs of all faculty, staff, and students regardless of location. Members of distance learning communities are entitled to library services and resources equivalent to those available in the traditional setting (ACRL Distance Learning Section Guidelines Committee, 2000).

Recent studies examining the needs of this unique and growing population show that services need to be designed to meet a wide variety of needs. Topping the list of requested services are reference, research, and instructional services. Reference services beyond phone calls include virtual reference (through chat and other digital means), choosing appropriate resources, document delivery of materials, and library instruction.

Many institutions have appointed or hired distance education or distance learning librarians to create and provide services to distance learners. These librarians are often one-person operations who function more as coordinators rather than full-service providers. Collaboration is the key to providing services to distance learning communities. Distance education librarians cannot offer reference services alone. This is especially true when services are offered more than forty hours a week. To be able to provide these services to remote learning communities, distance education coordinators or librarians need to form relationships with reference, informational, and instructional services librarians and staff. This article will focus on reference services offered to distant learning communities, and more importantly, the relationships that need to be built in order to offer reference and informational services to those faculty and students that are at a distance.

SERVICES TO DISTANCE LEARNING COMMUNITIES

The services that libraries offer, as we move further into the future, are quickly changing. Contrasting the various types of interactions taking place around a reference desk today with those of only 15 years ago, one sees evidence that a new millennium truly has dawned! The familiar activity at a reference desk of the 1980s was an in-person direct social interaction as compared to the various combinations of synchronous and asynchronous interactions in use today.

In the late 1980s, librarians usually communicated directly with people both face-to-face and on the telephone. If patrons were at a considerable distance and didn't need an immediate answer, they could write a letter. Of course, today those same three ways to perform reference services still exist; we have simply added to them.

Now that distant education has become a common method of teaching and learning, libraries are finding that the service options of e-mail and chat sessions are in demand. Tenopir and Ennis (2002) state, "Digital sources have brought about changes . . . in the type and range of resources available, and in the attitudes and expectations of reference librarians and patrons." During a typical two-hour desk shift, a reference librarian might check for e-mail questions several times, answer a toll-free phone number along with the regular phone, and see the occasional chat box pop up with questions. Tenopir and Ennis also tell us that today "we have more electronic reference services, but the same attention to personal interaction, whether online or in person, is still important." Computers are no longer only for looking up information; they are part of the total social interaction that allows librarians the ability to inform faculty, to teach students, and to collaborate with colleagues no matter where they live or work.

For each different format that a distant patron uses when asking questions, there are disadvantages. People needing immediate answers may wish to try a chat session. However, a chat session's disadvantage is that it can pop up (just as a phone call might come in) at a time when front-and-center patrons are at the desk needing our expertise. This added dimension can lead to the need for additional staffing.

At the reference desk, once the flow of on-site patrons slows down, the librarians can then turn their attention to the e-mail questions that have been accumulating. McClennen and Memmott (2002) point out, "It is imperative that the 'reference interview' represented by . . . an e-mail template or chat script be carefully designed to elicit enough information that the reference librarians can answer the patron's real question." However, the patron who is very happy using e-mail might find this process also less than perfect. Depending on the question and the process for answering, the actual reference interview might take several hours or even days to complete. This service will simply be too slow for many of the students who wait until the last minute.

If we were to return to the 1980s, mainly synchronous methods of delivery would be used for library instruction and reference services to any distant classes. Telnet and direct phone connections were the methods of reaching out to individuals and classes. Today we have added one new mode of synchronous instruction, the chat session. Librarians are now able to join a chat session and conduct group research instruction with or without the class's regular teacher. This instruction can take place whenever the class "meets," or it can be performed on an individual basis when needed. Librarians now are able to offer students the opportunity to ask questions when they, the students, need the answers. If there is a point in time when they want to ask a question and we are not available there is another option, this time there is an asynchronous connection, to reach us: e-mail.

The technology also allows libraries to offer web tutorials giving students the in-depth instruction they need when a quick answer just will not do. The average student with an in-depth question or needing instruction in the use of a particular database often feels more confident after talking to a "real" person. This is not always possible, and the use of these web tutorials makes it possible for instruction to happen anytime, anywhere. Many libraries are now using one of the most popular asynchronous methods for instruction to students at a distance (either in another part of the world or across the street).

In addition, the web tutorial lets the student "bone up" on research skills in their own time frame. The distance student of the new millennium is often non-traditional and may well have family and/or work obligations requiring them to think and study outside the box we usually think of as "study time."

The downside to the technology is that students at a distance may feel cut off from the confirming social experience of the physical reference desk and talking to librarians in person. The ramifications of this technology is that today's energetic librarian not only needs to know how to go about finding and supplying answers, how to explain the use of a full-text journal database, and how to translate the sometimes intricate processes of electronic reserves, she must also know something about trouble-shooting various technical aspects of access.

Finally, libraries also offer document delivery of non-electronic materials needed by our patrons. Materials, print and other formats, may be borrowed from libraries across the state, region, country, or world through a student's "home" library. The information needed for interlibrary loan can be provided through phone conversations, print forms, or even online. Distance students may also find that they need materials delivered from the home library to them. This means that different forms need to be designed, as the distance student will need to provide different information than traditional students. This use of varying forms will facilitate requests so that the student can receive needed materials as quickly as possible. However, during the busiest times of the semester, this delivery service can be (or at least can seem) very slow to our current online student generation.

These new technologies, however, enhance services offered to the distance student. E-mail, chat, library website tutorials, and toll-free numbers have all added to the richer texture of our modern library offerings. We can only imagine what another 15 or 20 years will bring!

ROLE OF THE DISTANCE EDUCATION COORDINATOR

According to the ACRL guidelines, libraries providing services to distance education students and faculty need to appoint a librarian-administrator or distance services librarian to coordinate services. These distance education librarians work in a variety of places in the library. Some libraries may place this librarian either in an access service or informational services department. More commonly, this librarian may function in a separate office as a one-person operation that makes providing services to a large distance education community difficult. Because one person cannot be everything to all people, the ability to work with a variety of people both in the library and outside of the library is extremely important for the distance education coordinator.

Often referred to as a "distributed model," the distance education librarian functions as a coordinator, not as service provider. Heller-Ross (1996) describes this model and the functions of the Outreach Information Services Librarian in her article. In the distributed model, the distance education librarian simply coordinates and develops services provided by a variety of entities throughout the library. The Interlibrary Loan Department provides document delivery; Information and Instructional Services provides reference and instruction; web services come from the Library's webmaster; and Circulation coordinates the electronic reserve materials. In order to offer services, especially reference, information and instructional services, these distance education librarians need not only to form relationships with the librarians and library staff in the reference and instructional areas of the library, but throughout campus and the distance learning community. Active leadership in heading up the program is a necessity for successful distance learning services. Being able to develop partnerships is the key to offering good services to the distance education learning community.

The librarian-administrator is minimally requested to do a variety of tasks in the ACRL guidelines. To provide adequate and relevant services and resources the distance education librarian should assess on a continual basis the needs of the distance learning community. It is recommended that a written profile of the community be created. This assessment can be done in a variety of ways including surveys, informal conversations, and feedback from the distance learning community. Communication and relationship building is very important in creating these profiles and determining what is needed by the users. The librarian coordinating the services needs the assistance of the reference staff that works with the students. Talking to the librarians working on the front lines with the users can be enlightening in terms of what services should be offered. The distance education librarian and the reference staff also need to form relationships throughout the distance learning community. The ability to talk and work with students to solve course-related and informational needs is an important part of designing and delivering effective services. According to Guenther (2001), "Combining all your remote user interactions–whether they occur by phone, e-mail, or the conclusions you draw from digital library usage statistics–is the key to developing the big picture view you'll need to provide effective services. None of these interactions taken alone gives the representative 'snapshot' of your remote user population."

Faculty teaching distance education courses cannot be ignored when determining the needs of the distance learning community. It is the instructors teaching the courses that determine the research and course requirements driving the student's information need. Usually when a student contacts the library, it is as a result of an imposed query initiated by the faculty member. Reference librarians and the distance education librarian need to work with faculty throughout the course cycle, often beginning with the creation of the course in order to integrate library-related activities and assignments, and ending with the evaluation of the course at the end. Communication and positive relationships with the faculty will assist in the creation of the profile of the needs of the distance education student.

The ACRL Guidelines stipulate that the Librarian-Administrator is asked to develop written statements of goals and objectives that are compatible with those of the administering library and institution as a whole. To accomplish this, relationships need to be formed with those individuals on campus that are responsible for directing and providing distance education opportunities. This may be a continuing education office, lifelong learning office, or a part of an academic department. Partnerships with these areas are essential in providing library services that support the educational needs of the distant learning community.

Collection development to meet the needs of the distance learning community is another area where the distance education librarian and subject bibliographers or selection librarians need to form relationships. Often these librarians are based out of the Reference Department and the distance education librarian needs to have a discussion with those selecting materials in order to determine the nature of courses being taught at a distance and the resources required. This communication will help insure that materials are purchased in a variety of formats to assist in meeting the needs of distance education students. Providing full-text resources and subject databases for the distant population is also important. When purchasing decisions are being made regarding electronic resources, the distance education offerings are an important element to consider. At times, duplicate or separate collections are purchased and housed at remote installations where large numbers of students reside. In this case, not only does the distance education librarian need to work with the appropriate bibliographer, but also with the library or institution that will be housing the collection. Relationships with those writing the collection development and acquisitions policies also need to be formed to make sure that the needs and profile of distance learning students are included in those policies.

CONCLUSION

The librarian coordinating services to distant students must build strong ties with various constituents both inside the library and outside, both within the profession and without. According to Kirk and Bartelstein (1999), "The most innovative approaches to changing the nature of higher education involve creative partnerships among academic and public librarians, computer professionals, college and university administrators, faculty, publishers, and venders." In order to reach successfully our students when and where they study or use the materials we make available, the person coordinating distance services must not only listen to and interact with the students, but also interact with the rest of the stakeholders. It is also important that there be an administrative presence supporting the services for distance learning and facilitating interactions.

The librarians and staff who work directly with students, the campus technology staff, the campus distant learning staff, the administrators, the professors and their staffs, and the staff in the library working with the library system make up the bulk of these stakeholders. The people on the front line handling the e-mail, fax, chat, toll-free and regular telephone questions are the reference librarians, the ones deciphering the "great tablets" of knowledge contained on the library's website. Anyone needing information not available electronically through the library's website, however, will probably have questions taking them through the library's document delivery system. Because of the impact that the document delivery system has on the complete distance service, the positive social and professional connections with those areas of the library are very important.

In order to be able to offer positive reference services to students who have hours beyond the normal, the reference desk and the distant services coordinator must become part of a greater world of distance librarians. As Richard Dougherty (2002) says, "With all the collaborative projects out there, libraries should not try to go it alone. Look for partnerships." The realm of reference consortia is now coming into existence.

For the last several years there have been many exciting murmurings about grouping together and linking around the world to offer "virtual librarians" with answers to any and all. The idea that librarians in Africa, India, Australia, and California could supplement those in Kansas (or Florida, etc.) is very seductive. This would offer the best service 24/7 without any of us actually staying up 24/7. Kansas is currently beginning its statewide linking of reference desks called KAN-Answer.

As today's librarians prepare for our futures in distance library services, we are reminded again that it is the connections and collaborations with people that make our jobs fruitful and rewarding. The social aspects of the reference desk do not go unnoticed. The people using our library in person see us, talk to us, smile, and help us feel that this is the best part of our jobs. Similarly this positive social relationship with our distance students (and distance faculty) is possible with today's technology. Fostering this positive relationship will bring them back often with more questions. The result will be that their papers and their projects will be filled with thoughtful research. Creating this atmosphere is not exclusively the distance services coordinator's job; it is everyone's job. We are all in academic libraries for the purpose of molding good students into good citizens and together we help them make possible the social connections that facilitate learning.

REFERENCES

ACRL, Distance Learning Section, Guidelines Committee. (2000), *Guidelines for Distance Learning Library Services*. Retrieved May 30, 2002 from http://www.ala.org/acrl/guides/distlrng.html.

Dewald, Nancy, Scholz-Crane, Ann; Booth, Austin; & Levine, Cynthia (2000), "Information Literacy at a Distance: Instruction Design Issues," *Journal of Academic Librarianship*, 26:1 (January), 33-44.

Dougherty, Richard. M. (2002), "Reference Around the Clock: Is It in Your Future?" *American Libraries* 33:5 (May), 44-46.

Guenther, Kim (2001). "Know Thy Remote Users," *Computers in Libraries*, 21:4 (April), 52-4.

Heller-Ross, Holly (1996), "Librarian and Faculty Partnerships for Distance Education," *MC Journal* 4 (Summer), 57-68. Retrieved November 18, 2002 from Wilsonweb Library Literature Fulltext.

Kirk, Elizabeth E. and Bartelstein, Andrea M. (1999), "Libraries Close in on Distance Education," *Library Journal*, 124:6 (April 1), 40-41.

McClennen, Michael and Memmott, Patricia (2001), "Roles in Digital Reference," *Information Technology and Libraries* 20:3 (September), 143-148. Retrieved November 8, 2002 from http://www.lita.org/ital/2003_mcclennan.htm.

Tenopir, Carol and Ennis, L. (2002), "A Decade of Digital Reference 1991-2002," *Reference and User Services Quarterly* 41:3 (Spring), 264-273.

Tenopir, Carol (2001), "Virtual reference services in a real world," *Library Journal*, 126:12 (July), 38-40.

Reference Beyond the Walls of the Library: Interacting with Faculty and Students in the 21st Century

Connie Ury
Carolyn Johnson

SUMMARY. The nature of research continues to evolve from accessing print publications in a library building toward retrieving information online, any time any place. Since patrons no longer need to enter a library building to access information, the social character of reference service has also changed. Demand for face-to-face reference interaction has declined, altering the traditional one-on-one venue for teaching information retrieval and evaluation. To develop new opportunities for influencing the information literacy levels of students, librarians at Northwest Missouri State University are creating outreach strategies that facilitate increased interaction with students and faculty. *[Article copies available for a fee from The Haworth Document Delivery Service: 1-800-HAWORTH. E-mail address: <docdelivery@haworthpress.com> Website: <http://www.HaworthPress.com> © 2003 by The Haworth Press, Inc. All rights reserved.]*

Connie Ury (E-mail: cjury@mail.nwmissouri.edu) is Library Outreach Coordinator and Lecturer and Carolyn Johnson (E-mail: carolyn@mail.nwmissouri.edu) is Information Librarian and Assistant Professor, both at Owens Library, Northwest Missouri State University, Maryville, MO 64468.

The authors would like to acknowledge the role of Joyce Meldrem as data compiler for the figures appearing in this article. Ms. Meldrem is Head Librarian for Collection Management and Assistant Professor, Owens Library, Northwest Missouri State University, Maryville, MO 64468 (E-mail: meldrem@mail.nwmissouri.edu).

[Haworth co-indexing entry note]: "Reference Beyond the Walls of the Library: Interacting with Faculty and Students in the 21st Century." Ury. Connie. and Carolyn Johnson. Co-published simultaneously in *The Reference Librarian* (The Haworth Information Press. an imprint of The Haworth Press. Inc.) No. 83/84, 2003, pp. 203-218: and: *Cooperative Reference: Social Interaction in the Workplace* (ed: Celia Hales Mabry) The Haworth Information Press. an imprint of The Haworth Press, Inc., 2003, pp. 203-218. Single or multiple copies of this article are available for a fee from The Haworth Document Delivery Service [1-800-HAWORTH. 9:00 a.m. - 5:00 p.m. (EST). E-mail address: docdelivery@haworthpress.com].

Digital Object Identifier: 10.1300J120v40n83_17

KEYWORDS. Reference outreach models, remote access, collaboration

INTRODUCTION

During the past five years, the authors have witnessed the alteration of reference services as information has become increasingly available without entering the library, and without asking librarians to facilitate access. University students and faculty no longer solely retrieve information by physically coming to the library to find sources published in print, archived or indexed on CD-ROMs, or stored on microform. Nor do they often request access to online databases available only through mediated searches conducted by librarians. Today, "a new generation of readers takes the Web for granted, expects to work online, and looks there for services" (Fleet and Sowards, 2001).

Even though Northwest Missouri State University students (FTE = 5,293, Fall 2002) are required to research information for class assignments and papers, the number of reference transactions at Owens Library has declined in the past ten years, especially after the World Wide Web became available through a GUI interface. Remote access to library databases has also increased. "Advances in telecommunications technology increasingly afford academic libraries the possibility of connecting their internal networks to the Internet and thereby offering university faculty, students and staff remote access to electronic resources and services" (Stanley and Lyandres, 2001). For example, forty-seven out of fifty-eight institutions of higher education, listed on Yahoo's directory (Yahoo!) for the state of Missouri, provide remote access to library databases.

REVIEW OF LITERATURE

The information environment is evolving from provision of in-house sources toward availability of online sources easily accessed from remote locations. Factors driving this change include a dramatic increase in the amount of information freely available via the Internet, the advent of commercial information providers, and the development of technology allowing remote access to library sources.

As early as 1999, Lipow documents trends supporting the assertion that demand for in-person, face-to-face reference service is decreasing because so much help is available via the Internet. She discusses a decreased demand for service at the reference desk, the public's view that the Internet is an adequate replacement for librarians' expertise, the struggle of reference librarians to stay up-to-date with the World Wide Web, and the availability of many commercial reference services on the Internet (Lipow, 1999). However, Lipow argues that much of what is available on the Internet lacks a high level of credibility and reliability. She also refers to Heckart's research that analyzes users' preferences regarding "human service vs. computer reference help" (Lipow, 1999). Heckart, writes Lipow, advocates that users believe they should be "self-sufficient in using computer systems" (Lipow, 1999) and thus do not ask librarians for help because they feel that asking for help is a sign of weakness. She concludes, "Reference service will rise only if it is as convenient to the remote user as a search engine" (Lipow, 1999).

Frank and Calhoun analyze the "Changing Nature of Reference Interaction" noting that "[i]nformation once restricted to a library building within prescribed hours is now often available from remote locations twenty-four hours a day" (Frank and Calhoun, 1999). They foresee a new role for reference librarians as that of "information consultants." They conclude that the "roles of the information consultant transcend the traditional boundaries of the classical library-bound professional who provided reactive reference services when approached. In direct contrast, consultants assume a proactive role, recognize and initiate consulting opportunities, and understand the importance of remaining in the 'information loop.' Although users have become more self-sufficient with the advent of electronic information, the consultant experiments with innovative ways to build relationships and provide services to clients and the larger university community" (Frank & Calhoun, 1999).

Tyckoson advocates, "Reference service will continue to change as our sources and technology change, but one-on-one personal assistance will remain its centerpiece" (Tyckoson, 1999). He contends that, due to the wide variety of formats in which information is currently available, patrons need librarians as guides more than ever before. If we accept the conclusion of Tyckoson that our expertise is essential, we must find ways to provide one-on-one personal assistance to users who interact with us online.

A year later, Wilson quotes Lipow when documenting that part of the trend toward online interaction has been due to the convenience offered by libraries' online presence via web pages available twenty-four hours a day, seven days a week. Wilson also attributes the popularity of remote access and requests for services to the anonymous nature of such an environment. Although e-mail requests may identify the initiator, they do not require face-to-face interaction. According to Wilson, this forum feels much safer for those who are uncomfortable with asking questions (Wilson, 2000).

Wilson calls for librarians to address this paradigm shift positively. He sets the stage, noting that "[t]he advent of the Internet has decisively altered the user culture, and has so decisively changed the relative importance of different user types, that no effort to reassert a traditional reference librarian role can possibly succeed" (Wilson, 2000). Consequently, librarians must find new ways to educate the public about the availability of information sources, teach users to discern the value of information, and anticipate the needs of patrons (Wilson, 2000).

In addition, Wilson concurs with Lipow that "reference statistics are decreasing in American academic libraries" (Wilson, 2000). He describes an environment in which "[m]any reference questions now come via individual reference librarian's e-mail, either from students seeking further assistance for classroom work or from faculty members who are on research leave or are working in their offices" (Wilson, 2000). Other changes involve the transference of service delivery from stationary reference desks to online mediums such as interlibrary loan via the library home page, e-mail reference service, and web-based checkout/renewal procedures designed to be used by patrons at remote locations. All of these functions were once performed in face-to-face transactions, but are now seamlessly available to remote users online. Wilson summarizes these changes, stating that "[i]n the post-Internet age of decentralized and distributed information resources, reference librarians no longer have a franchise as sole providers of information at the reference desk" (Wilson, 2000).

Anderson describes a transformation of the ways in which information is packaged in the early 21st century. Just because patrons don't enter the library doesn't mean that they don't have unanswered questions or a need to interact with those trained to act as guides to information sources. Anderson contends that librarians need to find new ways in which they can interact with users, especially those who are at remote locations (Anderson, 2001).

Trump, Tuttle, and Dugan agree that the demand for face-to-face reference service is declining. They speculate the following:

- Patrons are easily answering ready reference questions online via search engines or directories;

- Students hate to leave their computer for fear of "losing their seat" in overcrowded computer labs; and
- Access to information from remote locations causes users to forget that help is available since librarians are "out of sight, out of mind" (Trump, Tuttle and Dougan, 2001).

Dougherty describes the current climate of reference and information services. Based on data collected over a five-year period from his reference and change workshops, he notes that the job duties of information professionals are radically changing (Dougherty, 2002). Ten years ago, librarians spent the majority of their time answering in-person questions, delivering library instruction, and training patrons to manipulate indexes. Today, in addition to the duties described above, librarians are interacting with patrons online, publishing web pages, and creating online instructional materials. Dougherty suggests that librarians must move beyond complaining about the demise of traditional reference service and focus on developing new means for providing "value-added [digital] information services only available from trained and experienced librarians" (Dougherty, 2002).

Kyrillidou and Young, writing for the Association of Research Libraries in August 2002, document the following trends in research library public services between 1991 and 2001:

- Reference transactions in research libraries declined 21%, with the decline beginning in 1998.
- The number of students receiving library instruction increased by 41%, with each year showing an increase.
- Borrowing via interlibrary loan skyrocketed with a 109% increase and an average annual increase of 8.5%.
- Circulation of in-house materials declined 9%, with the decline beginning in 1996 (Kyrillidou and Young, 2002).

They conclude: "Higher levels of service activities in interlibrary loan and library instruction services indicate increased focus on providing access to, rather than ownership of, library resources. The declining trends of reference and circulation services since 1996 serve as indicators of the changing and increasing complexity of library users' reliance on electronic resources and services" (Kyrillidou and Young, 2002). These conclusions make sense when one considers that online access to many sources became readily available in 1996.

This article describes the outreach methods that the Owens Library Information Services Team (the reference department) uses to market and deliver reference services to all students and faculty who access information and conduct research from locations outside the library. These methods may be applicable in other libraries. Outreach activities include interaction via class web sites; research consultations; electronic reference service; print and online publicity; collaboration with faculty and student support service units; web-based resources for instruction and service; and online resources for research. Each of these initiatives is discussed in detail in the following sections.

MANAGEMENT BY FACT

The number of reference questions asked at Owens Library, Northwest Missouri State University, decreased 84% between the 1991-1992 and the 2000-2001 academic years (see Figure 1). The decline in reference questions began when a library instruction program was first instituted in 1991. The Northwest library instruction program includes course-embedded presentations for four general education classes, as well as upper level instruction upon request, and is marketed through personal contact, college meetings, and the library's web pages. The total number of students reached through library instruction presentations increased by 47% between the 1991-1992 and 2000-2001 academic years (see Figure 2). Although the direct impact of this instruction program on the demand for reference service cannot be proven, the decrease in reference desk traffic has continued as the instruction program matures. This trend supports the trends documented by the Association of Research Libraries in August 2002 for the years 1991 through 2001, showing a 21% decline in reference questions and a 41% increase in the number of students receiving library instruction (Kyrillidou and Young, 2002).

An additional factor impacting in-house reference service is the web presence of the library which, since the summer of 1996, has provided in-house and remote access to the library catalog; online databases; a wide range of research guides, webliographies, and bibliographies; as well as instructional materials. Owens Library Information Services Team members now author and maintain more than 400 web pages. Statistics for the web site were first generated for the 1997-1998 academic year. The Owens Library Home Page (Information Services Team, *Northwest Missouri State University Owens Library*, 2001) is

FIGURE 1. Reference Desk Questions 1991-2001

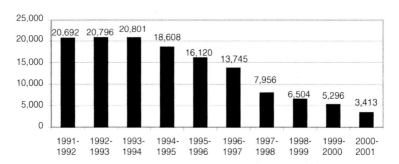

Data compiled by Joyce Meldrem, Head Librarian for Collection Management, Owens Library, Northwest Missouri State University.

FIGURE 2. Library Instruction Recipients 1999-2001

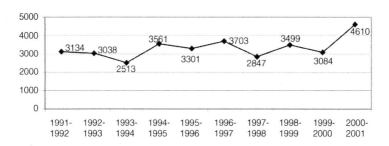

Data compiled by Joyce Meldrem, Head Librarian for Collection Management, Owens Library, Northwest Missouri State University.

the gateway that provides access to the library's web presence. Heavy use of this page is demonstrated by the more than 100,000 hits logged for it each year since 1997 (see Figure 3). Students use this front line resource to guide their research and information retrieval needs.

Since patrons were not coming to the library building with reference requests and information needs, librarians at Northwest Missouri State University decided to bring the library to them, through a variety of strategies and programs. In addition, since in-house reference transactions had declined to an average of 2-3 per hour, reference desk hours were cut to a minimum schedule: 9:00 a.m. to 12:00 noon and 2:00 p.m. to 5:00 p.m., Monday through Friday, and 6:00 p.m. to 9:00 p.m. on Sunday

FIGURE 3. Owens Library Home Page Hits 1997-2001

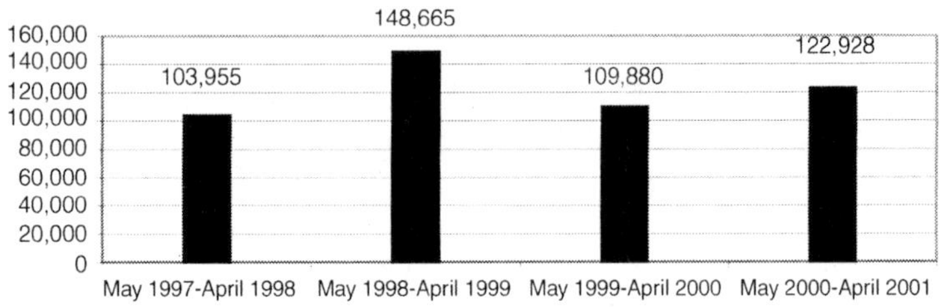

Data compiled by Joyce Meldrem, Head Librarian for Collection Management, Owens Library, Northwest Missouri State University.

(Saturday and Sunday afternoon reference traffic was exceedingly low). This gave reference staff the time and energy to sustain new and enhanced outreach efforts.

INTERACTING IN CLASS WEB SITES

In May 2002, the Information Services Team created a list of classes that include research by consulting the college catalog and from collective knowledge about previous course assignments. The course contact list was prioritized based on the level of research needed, the number of courses per college, and librarian expertise. Each librarian is contacting the instructor(s) of the classes they have chosen and offering to either provide library instruction or add library information to the class web site available via CourseInfo or Blackboard. As of November 2002, with less than half the contacts for the year completed, librarians had interacted with students or posted information via class web sites thirty times.

In addition, classes in which library instruction was previously delivered on-ground with supplemental web sites are now migrating to an online-only course format. Library instruction previously presented on-ground must now be reconfigured for online instruction. For the first time in Fall 2002, librarians interacted with online students via the class web site, participated in threaded discussions, and graded students' assignments in an online computer literacy course. Students learned advanced search techniques in specific web search engines and criteria for evaluating web sites. They were assigned to threaded discussion groups in which they collaboratively developed a search strategy to locate a web site about an assigned topic, selected a credible and reliable web site about the topic, and demonstrated in Microsoft Word documents how their web site fit each of five criteria (Authority, Design, Accuracy, Purpose, and Target) (Ury and Baudino, 2002). Librarians interacted with the student groups about searching and evaluation techniques via threaded discussions, downloaded the completed Microsoft Word documents, graded the students' work, and assigned student grades for the library component of the course module.

RESEARCH CONSULTATIONS

A research consultation service was initiated during the Spring 1992 term as an on-ground service. This service provides students with personalized, one-on-one research assistance by appointment where reference librarians discuss and demonstrate the use of recommended sources. Total uses of this service are documented by trimester in Figure 4. The popularity of this service has waned as the comprehensive library instruction program, which includes access points in four general education courses, has matured. The team began offering this service in an online format during the Spring 2002 trimester, as a service to students who are part of a growing online program (39 courses in Fall 2002) at the university. This service provides these students with personalized research assistance, a service formerly available only to on-site students.

ELECTRONIC REFERENCE SERVICE

E-mail reference service, via the Owens Library web page, has been available since Spring 1998. Students and faculty have not heavily utilized this service, even though there is a 24-hour turnaround time, Monday through Friday. Initially, discussions about providing a 24/7 chat reference service have not gone very far, since the Information Services Team currently has one position vacancy and we do not have funding to outsource virtual reference service. However, members of the reference staff have been intrigued by reports of the greatest amount of chat reference occurring during traditional (9 a.m.-9 p.m.) library hours (Maxwell, 2002), and may offer limited chat reference hours in the future if time and staffing permits.

FIGURE 4. Research Consultants Offered 1992-2002

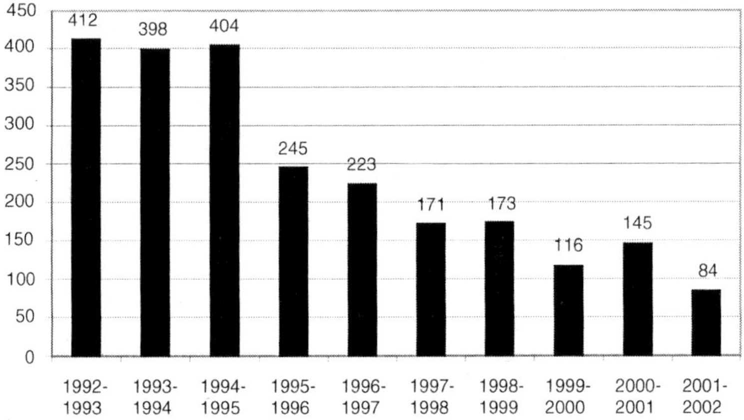

Data compiled by Joyce Meldrem, Head Librarian for Collection Management, Owens Library, Northwest Missouri State University.

MARKETING RESOURCES AND SERVICES

The Owens Library Information Services Team uses a variety of techniques to market library resources and services to patrons outside the library walls. For example, an e-mail news alert service for faculty was initiated in 2001. A "mass e-mail was sent to faculty and they signed up if they wanted to receive notices from the library about possible topics such as major changes in the library; new databases; new library Web pages; changes in current databases; and workshops offered. Eighty-five faculty members signed up to receive the service in Fall 2001. The first message included information about campus wide Web access to 'America: History and Life,' 'Education Full Text,' and 'CountryWatch.com' " (Information Services Team, *Annual Report* 2001). This service continues to provide the staff with a venue for contacting faculty. E-mail is also sent to all faculty members at the beginning of each trimester informing them of news and updates, as well as an opportunity to sign up to receive the e-mail alert service throughout the academic year.

Table tents were created in Fall 2002 to advertise a new library catalog and new database subscriptions. This model of outreach allows the Information Services Team to convey news to patrons across campus quickly. The table tents were displayed in the Student Union and other campus offices to reach users outside of the library building.

Librarians also reach students and faculty through newspaper articles and radio interviews. The publicity reaches a wide variety of clients and markets information about new services and databases. Both the campus and community newspapers have interviewed librarians and printed updated news several times in the past few years. Because all campus users log on to the university system with a unique user name and password, the campus is able to display "Notices of the Day" during the log-on process. The library has used this system for advertising library news when new services become available. These public venues enable wide dissemination of the information in a timely manner. When a new terminal server was brought up in Spring of 2003, the "Notices of the Day" feature will allow library news to reach remote, as well as on-campus students. Because of the new server, students and faculty will be able to access all library databases from any location using their university user name and password via a "Microsoft Windows Remote Desktop Web Connection."

In addition, "[d]uring Northwest faculty development days, librarians have offered Web page creation workshops, Internet and database searching techniques, and brainstorming sessions about Web-based curriculum materials" (Meldrem, Johnson, & Spradling, 2001). For more than five years, librarians have been guests at college and departmental meetings as each trimester begins. Members of the Information Services Team contact deans and department chairs to ask for five to ten minute blocks of time in which they can share information about new subscriptions and services from the library.

COLLABORATION WITH FACULTY

Librarians develop social relationships with students and faculty and make use of those contacts to disseminate information. Meldrem, Johnson, and Spradling describe Owens Library's collaboration with academic departments:

> Collaborative alliances can also be built through course development. Northwest librarians have taught both entire courses and modules within a course. For example, because a Northwest librarian taught Freshman Seminar (our freshman orientation course), the library staff was requested to assist in integrating

information research skills into the required freshman seminar curriculum. A library representative has also been added to the Freshman Seminar planning committee because of the contributions of this librarian. A similar experience occurred in Northwest's required general education computer literacy course. The computer literacy faculty recognized the benefits of consulting with the library staff in planning the course curriculum [after a librarian taught the course as adjunct faculty] and began consulting them and requesting their assistance on a regular basis in developing course materials. (Meldrem, Johnson and Spradling, 2001)

This type of partnership has also been extended to other areas. Several librarians enrolled in classes and participated in group projects with other students. One librarian acted as a research mentor for students enrolled in a humanities course, providing research consultations and tips, helping students convert research papers to web-based resources, and modeling an appropriate presentation format that highlighted works consulted in the presentation content.

Specific teams of reference librarians serve as departmental liaisons for four general education courses where course-embedded library instruction is delivered in both on-ground and online formats. Online tutorials have been developed in collaboration with departmental faculty for both an English composition and a speech course. Curriculum for a computer literacy course is continually refined as the Computer Science/Information Systems faculty and a team of three librarians evaluates and seeks to improve a performance-based small group exercise/threaded discussion.

Each reference librarian serves on at least one university committee. At meetings they network with campus faculty and develop collaborative relationships:

> University committee appointments are essential for improving visibility and fostering peer relationships between teaching faculty and library faculty. Even librarians who do not have faculty status can increase their visibility by participating in university committees in an ex-officio capacity. Conversations between colleagues can lead to enhanced understanding of student needs, assessment strategies, and instructional methods. (Meldrem, Johnson and Spradling, 2001)

Committee meetings are often the sites of initial contacts that lead to invitations to visit a class, become a teaching assistant in an online course, or participate in other faculty gatherings to share information. Librarians often share their research expertise when participating in groups such as computing access teams or student services groups. When librarians provide research-based information, faculty become accustomed to consulting them when information needs arise. Conversations in several team or group meetings have led librarians to develop web-based resources for faculty including a "Fair-Use Questionnaire" (Ury, 2002) that helps students and faculty understand the implications of plagiarism, as well as rubrics that faculty require students to complete when justifying the credibility and reliability of web sites for use in research projects (Mardis and Ury, 2002).

COLLABORATION WITH OTHER STUDENT SUPPORT SERVICE UNITS

Librarians at Northwest have a close working relationship with the Center for Information Technology in Education (CITE). For example, the Center's Curriculum Design Specialist recommends specific Owens' librarians, based on their subject expertise and interest, as resource consultants when developing new courses with online faculty. In addition, CITE links to the library's web page on their publicity CD; librarians attend technology workshops offered by CITE and teach copyright workshops for new online faculty; and librarians create webliographies about topics such as online assessment (Ury, 2001).

Librarians collaborate with the Freshman Seminar orientation program not only to develop and deliver introductory library instruction materials, but also to fine-tune instructors' assignments such as scavenger hunts. A freshman orientation career assignment is the result of a three-way collaborative effort that involves the Career Services Office, the freshman orientation faculty, and the Information Services librarians. In this assignment, students practice basic research strategies while evaluating their career choice or exploring career options.

WEB-BASED RESOURCES FOR INSTRUCTION AND SERVICE

Librarians at Northwest develop documents that address student needs, as indicated by faculty in conversational settings either at meetings or less formal gatherings. One such area is the development of web pages that provide examples for citing full-text online articles and web sites in MLA, APA, Turabian, and CBE style (Johnson, 2002). Faculty work in partnership with librarians as they review the examples available on the Owens Library home page, suggest changes or additional examples, and refer the Citing Sources web site to students.

The home page includes a link to database trials for faculty to evaluate and explore, as well as a "What's New" link (Information Services Team, *Northwest Missouri State University Owens Library*, 2001) that provides up-to-date information about new sources and resources available at the library or on the library home page. A "Faculty Services" web page (Johnson, 2002) has also been developed to provide information for faculty about library services and to enable them to quickly link to resources they need to use such as *Books in Print*. Finally, librarians provide one-on-one "Faculty Office Calls" (Johnson, 2001) for any faculty to help them incorporate library resources into their curriculum or to conduct their own research.

The Information Services Team provides a wide range of online tutorials and guides to enable students to develop appropriate research practices and information evaluation strategies. The "Owens Library Research" web page (Mardis, 2002) provides links to five online tutorials that are implemented as part of instruction in four general education library instruction access points. Additionally, the page links to learning objects that enable students to visually learn about research concepts. The "Find the Subject Database You Need" web page (Mardis and Wainscott, 2002) includes links to tutorials and guides for databases, some of which are produced locally. The "Course/Subject Resources: By Major" and "Course/Subject Resources: By Subject" web pages (Meldrem and Johnson, 2002) provide access to research guides, as well as annotated bibliographies and webliographies.

CONCLUSION

The reference environment no longer centers around a reference desk and face-to-face in-house questions and answers. As the information environment and information-seeking behavior continues to migrate to an online paradigm, the Information Services Team at Owens Library continues to seek new ways to interact with students and faculty who must be reached at locations distant from the library. The historical model of the library as a place where information is housed and librarians are available for consultations is no longer reflective of the reference service environment. The Team has learned to move beyond the walls of the library, both physically (in classes and meetings) and via print and online mediums to reach our patrons and provide guidance in information retrieval and source evaluation.

REFERENCES

Anderson, Charles R. (2001), "Reference Librarianship: A Guide for the 21st Century," *The Reference Librarian* 72, 5-20.

Dougherty, Richard M. (2002), "Reference Around the Clock: Is It in Your Future?" *American Libraries* 5, 4 (May) 44-46. Available from EBSCOhost Academic Search. EBSCO Publishing, accession no. 6611413. Accessed November 7, 2002, available from http://search.epnet.com/.

Frank, Donald G. and Calhoun, Katherine L. (1999), "The Changing Nature of Reference and Information Services," *Reference & User Services Quarterly* 39, no. 2 (Winter), 151-157.

Information Services Team (2001), *Northwest Missouri State University Owens Library*. Retrieved November 18, 2002 from the World Wide Web: http://www.nwmissouri.edu/library/.

Information Services Team (2001), *Owens Library Information Services Team Annual Report 2001*.

Johnson, Carolyn (2002), *Citing Sources*. Retrieved November 18, 2002 from the World Wide Web: http://www.nwmissouri.edu/library/citing/citing.htm.

Johnson, Carolyn (2002), *Faculty Office Calls*. Retrieved November 18, 2002 from the World Wide Web: http://www.nwmissouri.edu/library/services/officecalls.htm.

Johnson, Carolyn (2002), *Faculty Services*. Retrieved November 18, 2002 from the World Wide Web: http://www.nwmissouri.edu/library/services/faculty.htm.

Kyrillidou, Martha and Young, Mark (2002). Research Library Trends. Association of Research Libraries. Retrieved November 11, 2002 from the World Wide Web: http://www.arl.org/stats/arlstat/01pub/intro.html.

Lipow, Anne Grodzins. (1999), "'In Your Face' Reference Service," *Library Journal* 124, no. 13 (August) 50-53. Database online. Available from EBSCOhost Academic Search. EBSCO Publishing, accession no. 2140355. Accessed November 7, 2002, available from http://search.epnet.com/.

Mardis, Lori (2002), *Research*. Retrieved from the World Wide Web on November 18, 2002: http://www.nwmissouri.edu/library/courses/research/research.htm.

Mardis, Lori and Ury, Connie (2002), *Evaluating Websites: PART of the Research Process*. Retrieved from the World Wide Web on November 18, 2002: http://www.nwmissouri.edu/library/courses/evaluation/edeval.htm.

Mardis, Lori and Wainscott, Vicki (2002), *Find the Subject Database You Need*. Retrieved from the World Wide Web on November 18, 2002: http://www.nwmissouri.edu/library/articles/databases.htm.

Maxwell, Nancy Kalikow (2002), "Establishing and Maintaining Live Online Reference Service," *Library Technology Reports*, 38, no. 4 (July-August), 1-76. Database on-line. Available from InfoTrac Expanded Academic. Gale Group, accession no. A90307281. Accessed November 16, 2002, available from http://infotrac. galegroup.com/itweb/nwmosu_owens.

Meldrem, Joyce A. and Johnson, Carolyn (2002), *Course Subject Resources: By Major*. Retrieved from the World Wide Web on November 18, 2002: http://www. nwmissouri.edu/library/courses/majors.htm.

Meldrem, Joyce A. and Johnson, Carolyn (2002), *Course Subject Resources: By Subject*. Retrieved from the World Wide Web on November 18, 2002: http://www. nwmissouri.edu/library/courses/subjects.htm.

Meldrem, Joyce A., Johnson, Carolyn, and Spradling, Carol. (2001), "Navigating Knowledge Together: Faculty-Librarian Partnerships in Web-Based Learning," in *Library User Education: Powerful Learning, Powerful Partnerships*, edited by Barbara I. Dewey. Lanham: The Scarecrow Press.

Sowards, Steven W. (2001), "Declining that Invitation," *Reference & User Services Quarterly* 40, no. 3 (Spring), 209-213.

Stanley, Deborah and Lyandres, Natasha, (2001), "Reference Assistance to Remote Users," *The Reference Librarian* 73, 243-252.

Trump, Judith F., Tuttle, Ian P., and Dugan, Robert E. (2001), "Here, There, and Everywhere: Reference at the Point-of-Need," *Journal of Academic Librarianship* 27, no. 6 (November), 464-467. Available from EBSCOhost Academic Search. EBSCO Publishing, accession no. 5602724. November 7, 2002, available from http://search. epnet.com/.

Tyckoson, David A. (1999), "What's Right with Reference," *American Libraries* 20, no. 5, 57-64. Available from EBSCOhost Academic Search. EBSCO Publishing, accession no. 1835980. Accessed November 7, 2002, available from http://search. epnet.com/.

Ury, Connie and Baudino, Frank (2002), *Evaluating Web Sites*. Retrieved November 18, 2002 from the World Wide Web: http://www.nwmissouri.edu/library/courses/ usingcomputers/evalonline.htm.

Ury, Connie (2002), *Fair Use Questionnaire*. Retrieved November 18, 2002 from the World Wide Web: http://www.nwmissouri.edu/library/courses/copyright/ questionnaire.htm.

Ury, Connie (2001), *University Teaching Assessment Sources*. Retrieved November 20, 2002 from the World Wide Web: http://www.nwmissouri.edu/library/courses/ education2/ASSESSMENT.HTM.

Wilson, Myoung C. (2000), "Evolution or Entropy?" *Reference & User Services Quarterly* 39, no. 4 (Summer), 387-390.

Yahoo> Education> Higher Education> Colleges and Universities> By Region> U.S. States> Missouri. Retrieved November 7, 2002 from the World Wide Web: http:// dir.yahoo.com/Education/Higher_Education/Colleges_and_Universities/By_Region/ U_S_States/Missouri/Complete_List/.

Collaborate or Die!
Collection Development
in Today's Academic Library

James Cory Tucker
Jeremy Bullian
Matthew C. Torrence

SUMMARY. The practice of collection development faces many challenges in the present and likely future library environment. The following text presents concepts for collaboration as viable solutions to these challenges for collection development in academic libraries. In particular, a model of collaboration involving department faculty representa-

---

James Cory Tucker is Business Librarian, University of Nevada Las Vegas, 4505 Maryland Parkway, Box 457014, Las Vegas, NV 89154-7014 (E-mail: Cory.Tucker@ ccmail.nevada.edu). Jeremy Bullian is Librarian, Hillsborough Community College, Brandon Campus, 10414 East Columbus Drive, Tampa, FL 33619-7856 (E-mail: jbullian@hccfl.edu). Matthew C. Torrence is Instructor Librarian, University of South Florida, Tampa Library, 4202 East Fowler Avenue LIB 122, Tampa, FL 33620 (E-mail: torrence@lib.usf.edu).

[Haworth co-indexing entry note]: "Collaborate or Die! Collection Development in Today's Academic Library." Tucker, James Cory, Jeremy Bullian, and Matthew C. Torrence. Co-published simultaneously in *The Reference Librarian* (The Haworth Information Press, an imprint of The Haworth Press, Inc.) No. 83/84, 2003, pp. 219-236; and: *Cooperative Reference: Social Interaction in the Workplace* (ed: Celia Hales Mabry) The Haworth Information Press, an imprint of The Haworth Press, Inc., 2003, pp. 219-236. Single or multiple copies of this article are available for a fee from The Haworth Document Delivery Service [1-800-HAWORTH, 9:00 a.m. - 5:00 p.m. (EST). E-mail address: docdelivery@haworthpress.com].

Digital Object Identifier: 10.1300J120v40n83_18

tives and library liaisons is discussed. Consulting professional literature on this topic has offered insight into the establishment of librarian-faculty relationships, the process of collaboration, benefits of collaboration, as well as problems that may result from such cooperative relationships. Examples are illustrated from experiences at three academic libraries: University of Nevada Las Vegas, University of South Florida, and Hillsborough Community College. *[Article copies available for a fee from The Haworth Document Delivery Service: 1-800-HAWORTH. E-mail address: <docdelivery@haworthpress.com> Website: <http://www.HaworthPress.com> © 2003 by The Haworth Press, Inc. All rights reserved.]*

KEYWORDS. Collection development, collaboration, academic libraries, liaison, case studies

INTRODUCTION

For the foreseeable future it appears libraries and librarians will face many changes and challenges. Libraries must contend with new technology, decreasing budgets, increase in resource options, and rising prices of resources. These changes directly impact the collection development aspect of librarianship and create a more dynamic and challenging environment for the library profession. Perhaps more so than in the past, libraries will have to look beyond themselves and forge collaborative relationships with other entities in order to meet these challenges. Efforts made now toward this end will define the character of the profession and the perception and effectiveness of libraries for the future.

CHALLENGES

Academic libraries, like their counterparts in the public and private sector, are faced with increasing resource costs and decreasing budgets. Numerous articles have discussed these problems. According to the Library Materials Budget Survey (LMBS) by American Research and College Libraries (ACRL), in the 1990s "library materials base budgets did expand, but not as rapidly as in previous decades and certainly did not keep up with inflation for library materials" (Sewell, 2000). The LMBS study found that the overall average for the 12-year period (1986-1997) was 6.1% annually (Sewell, 2000). This trend does not appear to have changed in the years since the LMBS study.

In addition to library budget problems, there are concerns about the rising costs of library resources, most specifically serials. In a survey conducted by Born and Van Orsdel, results showed that "since 1986, the average annual increase in the serial unit cost for an ARL library was 8.8%." This increase amounted to a "total serial unit cost increase of 226%." In the last four years, the rate of price increases for serials is 10.4% and 9.0% in 1999 and 2000 and 8.3% and 7.9% in 2001 and 2002 (Albee & Dingley, 2001). In 1999-2000 "ARL libraries spent almost three times as much on serials" compared to 1986 and the "number of titles acquired was 7% fewer." The survey also found that journals are taking up an increasing amount of the libraries' acquisitions budget (2001). The straight-line projection shows that a journal which costs $125 in 1986 will cost $1,158 by 2012. In his 1991 article, Richard Dougherty sums up this dilemma, "In the short term, in spite of the existence of technology that scans, digitizes, and reproduces materials on demand, we are still very much at the mercy of major American and European publishers." In addition, monograph prices have also increased. The monograph unit cost has increased 66%.

Cost increases and budget cuts directly impact the collection development duties of the librarian. For the Collection Development Librarian the impact directly corresponds with collection management and selection and purchase of resources. The selection of resources will be even more difficult under these circumstances as the librarian will likely be forced to perform even more research on which serials to purchase, which, in turn, may require more research and selection of serial titles to cancel. Directly related to selection and deselection, the librarian may have to use various types of statistics including interlibrary loan requests, circulation statistics, photocopying frequency and citation analyses (Bustion & Treadwell, 1990). Under these circumstances, the librarian's job becomes more labor intensive.

In order to deal with these challenges, libraries and librarians must organize and employ collective strategies to help ensure the process of collection development is manageable. A "willingness to experiment" with strategies aimed at controlling costs is critical, according to Carpenter. "The national conversation has clearly documented the crisis in publishing, particularly the rapidly escalating prices of scientific, technical, and medical periodicals" (1996). Libraries must find ways to adapt in order to survive in an environment of ever-increasing materials costs and budget constraints.

SOLUTIONS

What can librarians and libraries do to overcome these challenges? From reviewing the literature, there are numerous options available for the library and the collection development librarian. One specific article by Lynden mentioned thirty different options for librarians. In the article, Lynden states "The approaches adopted by libraries to cope with the damaging effects of enormous increases in serial prices are wide ranging, using politics, on campus and off, budgetary techniques, and collection management strategies" (1992). The most common option to combat rising prices and lower budgets is for the library to enter some type of cooperative relationship, most often a consortia. Entering a consortia is usually the preferred method to combat these issues. Behind the basic principle of cooperation, however, is the concept of "give and take." The role of the consortia is indeed vital to the library's continued success. Yet the library should expect some loss of autonomy at the institutional level when entering into consortia relationships in return for an enhancement of library services. This likelihood will require a "new world view" from the entire library staff concerning collaborative approaches on this scale (Carpenter, 1996). There are opportunities, however, at the university level where libraries can forge collaborative relationships.

In an article by Wicks, Bartolo and Swords, "Another type of cooperation in collection work is that of the professional bibliographer and the departmental faculty" (2001). Libraries have the ability to develop relationships with academic departments throughout the university. Libraries can enlist the aid of academic departments to ease the impact of rising costs and budget cuts. As with consortia, in collaboration with academic departments, "it is critical that participants understand the importance, purpose, need and permanence of collaborative collections management" (Hightower & Soete, 1995). Chu notes in his 1995 study on collaboration in a loosely coupled system of librarian and faculty relationships, that collaboration can be problematic due to a "lack of understanding of the purpose of collaboration." In addition to well-defined lines and levels of communication, Chu states "the substance of communication," or the "content and procedures of collection development" must be clearly understood by the collaborating partners (1995). Though it may seem logical that substantive communication is necessary to ensure successful cooperative relationships, the professional literature has repeatedly shown a deficiency in communicating the expectations of collection development between librarians and faculty. The onus for relating the "substance" of collection development should rest on the librarian. After all, in a librarian-faculty member relationship, it is the librarian who has primary responsibility for the library collection. It may be in the faculty member's best interests to collaborate, but realistically the library collection will remain secondary to teaching, research, and other responsibilities demanded by the individual's department.

To further complicate the collaboration process, faculty often do not have the bibliographic experience required for materials selection (Drummond et al., 1991). One way Drummond et al. suggests to counter this particular knowledge gap is to hold "seminars or workshops sponsored by the library" (1991). Implementing an annual workshop near the start of the academic and/or fiscal year would provide an opportunity for new faculty liaisons to learn what is required of them in the collaborative relationship. Participating faculty and librarians could also use these workshops to define their cooperative affiliations for the rest of year.

BENEFITS OF COLLABORATION

Collaborating with academic departments is a mutually beneficial process. First, it helps librarians with their job of managing and selecting resources for the collection. Managing and selecting resources is the most time consuming aspect of collection development. Faculty and staff in academic departments can help the librarian with making these difficult decisions, saving time and money. Decisions involving new materials, especially in the electronic medium, are now subject to multiple forms of collaboration. This involves more than just implementation, as pointed out by Carpenter in her article (1996) about collaboration and competition. The following quote illustrates this point quite well in espousing that, " . . . deciding to subscribe to an index in one of its electronic formats rather than in print requires the traditional assessment of scope and coverage, timeliness, index access points, and cost. This decision also demands a careful consideration of current and future networking capabilities, proposed access sites, number of simultaneous user licenses required, and level of customization required to meet local system requirements. These decisions often cannot be made with the knowledge base of the library liaison and the faculty representative; in these situations, the systems or technology unit of the library or information center must be involved in the decision to negotiate the above elements, as well as providing final installation."

Second, building relationships with academic departments can open the door for collaborative purchasing of library resources. Besides being a resource for advice, these academic departments can be a great source of funds. As in the case of libraries, academic departments are provided a set amount of funds. Like libraries, academic departments have seen their budgets shrink. Being researchers, they also understand about the rising costs of library resources. This provides an excellent environment to foster a collaborative relationship in collection development. By sharing the cost of library resources, libraries and academic departments will be able to not only keep current resources, but add vital new resources. This assures and perhaps expands on an adequate base of resource materials (Hightower & Soete, 1995). Keeping current resources while adding new materials will have a positive impact on student and faculty research needs.

A third, qualitative, byproduct can be achieved through collaboration. A strengthening of the academic environment within the institution can result from the communicative process between faculty and librarians. Furthermore, collaboration can foster a degree of understanding between the faculty sphere and the librarian sphere. The librarian and requisite faculty liaison(s), in effect, act as a support structure linking the library to the academic department(s). If, as Drummond, Mosby and Munroe note, "the continued progress of the library facilitates progress in the scholarly community," the converse would also seem to apply in that the scholarly community can be affected adversely by deficiencies of the library. The authors continue by stating "while scholars often do not have a clear picture of the needs of the library, librarians often do not know enough about the scholarly environment" (1991). As it is essential for the librarian to communicate the library's expectations of the faculty, it is equally important for the library to know the faculty's expectations. The process of collaboration can bridge the gap between separate academic spheres and promote a greater understanding of the scholarly environment encapsulating them both and the needs required to support this environment.

These examples illustrate how cooperation can be beneficial to both parties. Knoche agrees "cooperative arrangements often enable user expectations to be addressed in a cost effective manner, and the resulting increased customer satisfaction and savings in real dollars and staff time also positively impacts staff morale" (1999). These circumstances illustrate the fact that collaboration within the university has many benefits.

However, the process of collaboration is not an easy one. It takes time and effort to build relationships through communication and marketing.

COLLECTION DEVELOPMENT PROCESS

Collaboration is, of course, dependent on the method of collection development chosen (or evolved) by the academic institution. There are abundant grades and infinite levels between them, but as described by a trusted colleague at the University of South Florida (USF), there seem to be three basic levels of collaborative collection development. The first involves little or no control by the librarians with the funds and decision-making process largely in the hands of the departmental faculty. In this method, librarians still have some influence, but the authority lies with the colleges and influential administrators. The second level, not surprisingly, utilizes opinions and decision-making abilities of subject-based librarians and their faculty and department liaisons to make purchases and collection-based decisions. This method is employed by USF and other universities and colleges as an excellent means to better the collection, as well as foster an increase in scholarly communication. The third method sees control largely in the hands of specific collection development librarians and subject bibliographers, whose job assignment and focus it is to shape and monitor the collections on behalf of the university and the departments.

To restate, though, most academic libraries are somewhere in between each of these descriptions. In libraries with the funds and staff to employ dedicated collection development librarians, there is still communication with the faculty as part of their task; the control rests in their hands and outside the department, but the influence and guidance of the faculty must still be felt. Likewise, the systems of allocation under almost entirely departmental control must still rely on the librarians for some information regarding the collection, even if it relates almost entirely to physical and clerical matters. The "method in the middle," or the most collaborative approach(es), must therefore employ the best combination of these factors to support effective collection management.

PROCESS OF COLLABORATION

As with consortia agreements, many principles such as, building relationships and managing relationships are important when collaborating with academic departments. Librarians will have to realize that the collaboration processes are "not static, but rather dynamic processes which constantly evolve" (Knoche, 1999). Concerning organizational relationships Knoche points out "most organizational relationships emerge slowly and incrementally, gradually strengthening and expanding as successes accrue and trust emerges." Knoche also states that "the relationship builds a history and set of norms, providing stability and predictability to the relationship" (1999). For librarians, collaboration revolves around relationship building and communications. The collaboration process starts with building relationships with each academic department. The process begins with communicating with academic departments through liaison work and library marketing. The building of these collaborations and their effectiveness will depend on previous dealings with the library and the library liaison.

Liaisons are the key communicators to the faculty and academic departments. Liaisons are on the "front-line" for the library building relationships. Subject Liaisons market library services and resources to their specific academic departments. They are building a "working" relationship with these departments. In speaking of communication Lynden states, "A very significant part of the budget process is communication. . . . First, the library needs to explain the situation (library funding) to faculty, students, staff, alumni and friends. There is a price crisis and it needs to be understood by the community" (1992). Liaison work begins by establishing an interpersonal relationship with each faculty member. Knoche states, "Although transactions originate primarily for reasons of economic exchange, as members get to know one another, they soon become enmeshed and embedded in the social interchanges that transpire: the abstract becomes personalized, friendships develop, and individuals engage in mutual support" (1999). According to the author, "Studies have also determined that personal relationships are a crucial factor in the decision-making process. When attempting to make a sound decision, people tend to conduct business with those familiar to them" (Knoche, 1999).

As shown above, developing a good working relationship with academic departments helps start a collaborative effort in the university. Lynden states, "The education of the faculty members to the concerns of the library is imperative" (1992). Starting a line of communication through marketing can help build a collaborative relationship with academic departments. Lynden agrees, "Constant communication with university departments and the library can result not only in improved relations, but also some cooperation. We must encourage departments to include library acquisitions in their next grant proposal. Or the department, understanding the inability of the library to support a new area of research may offer to supplement the Library's allocation with [a] departmental fund" (1992). The key to communication involves understanding the needs of both the library and academic departments. With liaison work, marketing by the library as one entity is important. Like subject librarians, the library must continue the communication process aiming its marketing efforts to the entire university including faculty and students. There are many ways in which the process can be made more efficient, and more effective communication, if not more communication in general, would seem an obvious method. The expenditures of ARL libraries for 1996-97 demonstrate a shift of monies from monographic to serial resources and the overall shift from 1986-1997 is even more telling; during this period, serials spending doubled, but an average of 6% fewer titles were purchased (Wolf & Bloss, 1998). This demonstrates the need for increased communication, of the efficacy thereof, between the faculty and their library representatives in order to manage these new cost-based challenges. Consortia arrangements offer increased buying power, but the needs of each college, university, and department must still run at the front.

Another important method related to this increased communication is the role of the user. In reviewing sources for this article, frequent mention was made to the library user as an important element in the collaborative method of collection development. As written by Carpenter, "Library users should play an important role in our planning and choices" (1996). Others have noted this as well and though it seems apparent that this is true, academic departments cannot be truly involved until they understand what they already have at their disposal and the effect they can have on the collection itself (Wicks et al., 2001). This, too, may seem another all too obvious point, but there may be potential for each and every academic library to increase the formality of student involvement in the collection development and management process.

Students today are inherently more aware of the new library materials, especially due to the explosion of the Internet and new methods of publishers in distributing their new materials and products. While it is often true that libraries aren't aware of a need until a patron comes looking for a product we don't own, publishers are now distributing notice of these sources and products directly to faculty and students via professional associations, journals, direct communication, and even the online catalog (Eckman & Quandt, 1995). At USF, for example, OPAC searches provide a listing of results that start with the most recent, and often in-process or on-order items. In this way, students are serendipitously exposed to new studies and research, even if it is at the expense of many a cataloger besieged with rush-catalog requests because the patron looked no further than the first few entries for newly published materials. Librarians may see this type of interaction, and the direct contact by publishers to faculty, change their role somewhat, but it will also allow the departments to engage in discussion and debate over new products before the librarian has had to make a purchase decision.

The role of the collection development librarian, especially in the collaborative environment, is also shaped greatly by perspective. Research and study in the field brought to the forefront an often-overlooked aspect of this perspective, the "anticipation of needs" or the "eventual rather than the immediate" (Chu, 1995). In his study of librarian faculty relationships, Chu states that when abundant, an approval plan is an excellent method to ensure that the needs of the libraries are met by the collection, but that the two sides of the coin are responding to different pressures and using their communication and collaboration in different ways (1995). The following quote sums up these perspectives quite well by articulating, " . . . librarians respond to factors such as institutional budget constraints that result from state legislative action or price increases from publishers above the rate of inflation. At the same time, other parties in the relationship, the academic departments, try to respond to demands from accrediting agencies and employers for their graduates" (Chu, 1995). Most librarians, at one point or another, have faced this challenge, but it must be recognized for an effective undertaking of any collaborative collection management initiative.

The marketing and liaison work demonstrate the painstaking process of collaboration. Knoche agrees "collaboration rarely happens by accident, but rather is a process which requires deliberate effort on the part of individuals at all levels" (1999). This point was also supported in interviews by Chu. He found that "both faculty and librarians see the system as a method of cooperation, but stress that it must be a two-way street" (1997).

EXAMPLES OF COLLABORATION

To provide illustrations of the effectiveness of collaborative relationships with academic departments, examples of collaborative efforts at

Hillsborough Community College, University of Nevada, Las Vegas and the University of South Florida will be described.

University of Nevada, Las Vegas

At the University of Nevada, Las Vegas, there are several examples of collection development collaboration. These examples illustrate using funds from both library and academic departments to purchase new resources. During my initial correspondence with the College of Business, there was a repeated inquiry concerning the purchase of *Lexis-Nexis Academic Universe*. At the time, the library did not have a subscription to *Academic Universe*, however, the College of Business and the College of Hotel Administration did have a 4-station subscription for *Academic Universe*. The College of Business purchased three stations and Hotel Administration one station. The four terminals were located in a computer lab at the College of Business. The subscription had several limitations. Faculty and students had to physically visit the lab to access the database. Remote access was not available. The computer lab was only open for a specific time period. In addition, there were other limitations, such as limits to printing and e-mailing. The total cost of the subscription at the time was $7,200 or $1,800 per station.

After building a relationship with the Dean of the College of Business and Chairs of each department, the library approached the College of Business and the College of Hotel Administration concerning a collaborative effort to buy university access to *Academic Universe*. Both departments agreed to an annual donation of $7,200 towards the purchase of the database. The library paid the remaining balance and in a couple of months the University had *Academic Universe*.

Another example of collaborative collection development was the purchase of the Securities Depository Center (SDC) database (Mergers and Acquisitions). Dr. Sam Choi, Chair of the Finance Department, approached the Library about chipping in to buy this database. He had secured funding from the College of Business and the Library at the William S. Boyd School of Law. He still required $500 to purchase the database. At the time, Lied Library did not have much funding because it was near the end of the fiscal year. However, Lied Library discovered available funds in an Endowment for Finance, but it still did not cover all of the expense. Looking at available funds, it was discovered that the Economics Department also had an endowment with a significant amount of funds. Dr. Choi and the Business Librarian called the Chair of Economics, Dr. Stephan Miller, and proposed a plan for the Economics Department to chip in the rest of the money. Dr. Miller agreed because it is a useful resource for his faculty and the database was purchased.

The rewards and efforts of collaboration are best described in an e-mail from Dr. Choi, "I appreciate your efforts to acquire the databases including *Lexis/Nexis*. In particular, I loved your attitude shown to us in my last department meeting that nothing is impossible if we all work together, in response to the skeptical view on the data acquisition. Thank you very much."

University of South Florida, Tampa

The University of South Florida (USF) also exhibits a classic example of one of the many methods of collaborative collection development. Along with a large percentage of colleges and universities nationwide, USF employs a fairly traditional approach that involves library liaisons engaging in regular and formalized contact with representatives from the academic units and departments. These assignments ideally encompass areas of subject specialization for the librarians, or at the very least, areas of interest and study. By combining (relatively) specialized librarians with faculty in each unit, the responsibilities are shared and, as noted by Wicks et al., in her study of the liaison program at the Kent State Libraries, "The Library and the University successfully turned a large undertaking into a manageable and mutually beneficial process" (2001).

As with any system that represents, and survives on, scholarly communication, there are numerous hurdles to this type of symbiotic relationship. A number of articles have addressed the reduction in library budgets, with some going on to assert a drastic decline in the overall buying power of libraries over the last ten years (Branin et al., 2000). This buying power must also be scattered among the different colleges, and then the departments themselves must compete for "funds within funds," so to speak. As noted by the literature, a "formula allocation" that takes into account the number of students, average cost of materials, and importance in the university hierarchy of research focus in determining each slice of the pie (Wicks et al., 2001). Despite these ratios, the very essence of different methods of scholarly communication, as asserted by Branin et al., are at the root of many problems related to collaborative collection management (2000). As all librarians are aware, and as these authors succinctly stress, some fields of study communicate primarily with journals and serials publications, while others focus on monographs or even electronic materials (2000). These different types of demands, and the varying cost of titles from discipline to discipline can lead to consternation and conflict over perceived inequity. An example of this is provided by Felix Chu in his earlier article on collaboration and loosely coupled systems. In his study, he spoke with a representative in home economics asked to cut a budget that totaled less than $5,000 to keep a group of important physics titles whose price had increased over $2,000 (1995). This request was made with these important core titles in mind, but what of the 300 majors in home economics compared to only 34 undergraduate and graduate students in physics (Chu, 1995)? The opinions of multiple faculty, departments, and liaisons would all need to come together to weigh the relative importance of such decisions and the reductions that must be made. This is not unlike what many libraries, including USF, have faced when unpleasant decisions, or the possibilities thereof, raise their ugly heads.

USF faced a similar challenge related to the budget, as have most academic libraries across the country. Faced with the prospect of a possible drastic budget reduction, the Division of Collections implemented a Serials Review Project to rate the importance of serial titles subscribed to by the Tampa Library. The participation of the liaisons, and indeed, all interested faculty, was absolutely integral to the success of this project. Even ignoring bundled and electronically purchased titles, which are much harder to renegotiate and affect the contracts thereof, rating the "traditional" print titles according to research and curricula importance could not have been accomplished without each of the subject librarian liaisons contacting and engaging in conversation with their respective departmental counterparts. Fortunately for all involved, the cuts to the budget did not force truly difficult decisions (as of yet), but preparation is priceless in these situations and effective collaboration helped avoid the lack of faculty voice in the trimming process, as well as the elimination of desired resources over less-desired ones.

Hillsborough Community College, Tampa, FL

Having first garnered collection development experience working at a university library, this author has found that the collection development responsibilities at Hillsborough Community College, Brandon Campus (HCC-BR) have proved to be quite a challenge. No longer one of many with responsibility over a collection, rather now I am one of two librarians employed at the Brandon Campus Library (BLIB). Between us is shared the burden of maintaining and developing the entire collection. Proportionally our library collection (17,300 titles) is significantly smaller than an average university library's. But collection development isn't merely about quantity. The primary focus should rest on the quality of the collection. One of the biggest hurdles thus far has been providing quality selection for the large variety of subjects needing representation in the library. But as the collection development position also includes a myriad of other duties including reference responsibilities, bibliographic instruction, and committee work to name a few, there is only so much time to spend pouring over book reviews and selection materials. Trying to keep abreast of current materials required to represent the entire college curriculum has been a futile pursuit.

BLIB is no different than most libraries in the present economy, in that the budget is hardly sufficient to maintain a quality, prospering collection of both traditional and electronic materials. Instead of bemoaning the general state of library collection budgets, local budgetary characteristics will be described. HCC has four main campuses, each with a library/learning resource center. From the budget allocation to the campus libraries, which varies year to year, immediately off the top comes funding for standing orders, periodicals, and electronic database subscriptions. Whatever is left is then divided among the libraries according to full-time enrollment (FTE) figures. Simply put, the larger the FTE for a campus, more money is available for the campus library. Unfortunately for our library, Brandon Campus does not have the largest FTE of HCC's four campuses.

Given the limiting factors of time, expertise, and funding illustrated in the previous paragraphs, it didn't take long to realize the need to solicit some form of collaborative approach in regards to collection development. Faced with these collection development challenges, the two librarians found two approaches which have had varying degrees of success.

Previous to our arrival at HCC-BR, there was no system in place for faculty collaboration with the library for collection development purposes. In lieu of an established system, our two librarians began using opportunities such as Faculty meetings, e-mail postings, personal interaction, and even the "Faculty Handbook" for library services to encourage faculty participation. This intermittent, personal approach has resulted in collaborative relationships with a number of faculty members. Through them the library has received input on (and on the rare occasion departmental funding for) specific materials, in both traditional and electronic forms, needed in the library to support class curricula. The HCC-BR faculty, however, includes a majority population of adjunct or part-time faculty members. For the current 2002-03 academic year there are 123 part-time faculty (minus dual enrollment faculty) employed at the Brandon campus versus only 46 full-time faculty (including the two campus librarians). As it is, my colleague and I have only cemented collaborative relationships with a small percentage of our full-time faculty. Adjuncts do not attend faculty meetings and their part-time status is a limiting factor on their availability for contact on and off campus, as well as their participation in faculty issues. Until we are able to implement a system such as a faculty/librarian representative model that incorporates input from entire faculty departments including adjunct faculty, we will not truly experience the benefits of faculty collaboration.

Sometimes, however, collaboration can come from unexpected sources. This was indeed the case when BLIB embarked on a collaborative relationship with our campus Student Government Association (SGA). The SGA has proved to be an extremely beneficial resource for the campus. Their funds have been made available to support student-centered activities, resources, and other objectives. It is through SGA, and it's Student Activities Advisor, Dr. Earl Paul, that BLIB received funding for a rather robust "leisure reading" collection. Funded entirely by SGA, the leisure collection is comprised of hardback books supplied through a McNaughton Book Lease Plan and a paperback book section. In our second year of the agreement with SGA, they have funded approximately $1,800 per year to support the lease book service. Additionally, SGA has funded periodic spending sprees at a local, chain bookstore to develop our paperback book collection of popular titles in a variety of genres. To date, we've made three trips, purchasing $1,040 in paperback books with an additional $612 allocated for purchase of paperback display racks. This leisure collection has proven to be a popular addition to the library among students, faculty, and staff alike. Furthermore, it is a concrete example of how mutual benefit can be achieved through collaborative relationships.

OTHER FORMS OF COLLABORATION

These examples clearly show that collaboration works well in the academic environment. Collaboration can help the library more efficiently perform collection development and can help the library add resources to its collection. This is all good news, but collaboration should not stop here. There are other projects related to collection development which libraries and academic departments may collaborate. One specific example is Scholarly Publishing and Academic Resources Coalition (SPARC). It has been three years since SPARC was launched by the Association of Research Libraries (Albanese et al., 2001). Libraries and academic departments can collaborate by purchasing SPARC resources. In addition, libraries and academic departments can take the initiative and collaborate by creating SPARC resources. Libraries can be their own solution to rising costs and shrinking budgets.

POTENTIAL ROADBLOCKS

As with any process, there are potential problems to look for when collaborating with academic departments. According to Chu, "One crucial component to lateral relationships in many educational institutions is the availability of resources. The units within the institution must compete with each other for portions of the finite resources" (1997). Chu brings up a great point. Although libraries and academic departments can collaborate to purchase resources, they both are competing for funding from the university. With decreasing budgets, this competition for funds will continue to be fierce and could hamper collaborative efforts.

In addition to university funding, another potential problem is commitment. When sharing the cost for resources, librarians and academic departments must deal with the issue of commitment. Will the agreement be permanent, every few years or annual? There are potential problems with trust and economic factors that may cause the library or department to back out of a deal.

Another problem is ownership. If a resource is purchased through collaboration, who owns the material? This may be an issue that could be settled by percentage of monetary output. However, this issue needs to be addressed before the materials are purchased.

A final problem is monetary flow or "red-tape." Libraries and academic departments have separate accounting systems, although all payments usually flow through the university's disbursements office. Each university department has separate accounts and paperwork can be an issue. Many times payments from separate accounts can slow the process of purchase or renewal. A system must be established to offset any potential inefficiency in the accounting system.

CONCLUSION

Collaboration can help libraries conquer rising resource costs and shrinking budgets. Whether the process involves other libraries or academic departments, collaboration can be an important tool. Libraries must explore this avenue, making this a priority for the future. Using subject librarians, through liaison and marketing, libraries can build effective monetary relationships with academic departments. These relationships can be very effective but "in order to be successful, collaboration must involve not only the exchange of resources, but a commitment which embodies the mutually beneficial relationships" (Knoche 33). Libraries and librarians must acknowledge that building relationships is a time consuming process that may take several years. In the long run, the efforts should pay off.

REFERENCES

Albanese, A., Berry, J., Bryant, E., Oder, N., and Rogers, M. (2001), "Looking Back, Looking Ahead," *Library Journal* 126(20), 72.

Albee, B. and Dingley, B. (2002, June), "U.S. Periodical Prices–2002," *American Libraries Online* Retrieved August 7, 2002 from <http://www.ala.org/alonline/archive/periodicals02.html> Born, K. and Van Orsdel, L. (2001), "Searching for Serials Utopia," *Library Journal* 126(7), 53-58.

Branin, J. J., Groen, F. K., and Thorin, S. E. (2000), "The Changing Nature of Collection Management in Research Libraries," *Library Resources and Technical Services* 44(1), 23-32.

Bustion, M. and Treadwell, J. B. (1990), "Reported Relative Value of Journals versus Use: A Comparison," *College & Research Libraries* 51, 142-151.

Carpenter, K. H. (1996), "Competition, Collaboration, and Cost in the New Knowledge Environment," *Collection Management* 21(2), 31-46.

Choi, S. (2002, February 14), "SDC Database," personal e-mail to James Cory Tucker accessed 14 February 2002.

Chu, F. (1995), "Collaboration in a Loosely Coupled System: Librarian-Faculty Relations in Collection Development," *Library and Information Science Research* 17, 135-150.

Chu, F. (1997), "Librarian-Faculty Relations in Collection Development," *The Journal of Academic Librarianship* 23, 15-20.

Drummond, R. C., Mosby, A. P., and Munre, M. H. (1991), "A Joint Venture: Collaboration in Collection Building," *Collection Management* 14(1/2), 59-72.

Eckman, R. H. and Quandt, R. E. (1995), "Scholarly Communication, Academic Libraries, and Technology," *Change* 27(1), 34-44.

Hightower, C. and Soete, G. J. (1995), "The Consortium as Learning Organization: Twelve Steps to Success in Collaborative Collections Projects," *The Journal of Academic Librarianship* 21, 87-91.

Knoche, C. M. (1999), "Critical Factors for Collaboration in an Academic Library Setting," *Advances in Library Administration & Organization* 16, 31-94.

Lynden, F. C. (1992), "Strategies for Stretching the Collection Budget," *Journal of Library Administration* 16(3), 91-110.

Sewell, R. G. (2000, August), " 'Big Heads' Library Materials Budget Survey Now on ARL Website," *A Bimonthly Report on Research Library Issues and Actions from ARL, CNI, and SPARC* 211. Retrieved September 12, 2002 from <http://www.arl. org/newsltr/211/lmbs.html>.

Swaine, C. W. (1999), *Paving the Way for Collaboration Between Librarians and Faculty*. Virginia: Old Dominion University. (ERIC Document Reproduction Service No. ED 437958).

"The Impact of Serial Costs on Library Collections," (2001, October), *ARL Bimonthly Report* 218. Retrieved September 29, 2002 from <http://www.arl.org/newsltr/218/ costimpact.html>.

Wicks, D. A., Bartolo, L., and Swords, D. (2001), "Four Birds with One Stone: Collaboration in Collection Development," *Library Collections, Acquisitions, and Technical Services* 25, 473-483.

Wolf, M. T. and Marjorie E. Bloss, M. E. (1998), "Without Walls Means Collaboration," *Information Technology and Libraries* 17(4), 212-215.

If They Build It Will They Come?
Cooperation and Collaboration to Create a Customized Library

Barbara J. D'Angelo

SUMMARY. The core mission of Arizona State University (ASU) East Library is electronic delivery of resources and services accompanied by a strong commitment to personalized service and to facilitating the campus educational goals through cooperative and collaborative partnerships with faculty and programs. The Library and the Multimedia Writing and Technical Communication Program (MWTC) have developed and implemented an instructional program in information skills and system design. The MWTC Program emphasizes information access, management, and design as some of the primary skills taught. The Program's applied nature attempts to give students as much practical experience as possible in environments which approximate the workplace. The Library-MWTC partnership combines the expertise of the Library and the faculty to meet the educational goals of the Program in a real-world setting by facilitating the creation and design of a customized MWTC library information system. The faculty and librarian are collab-

Barbara J. D'Angelo is Reference/Instruction Librarian, Arizona State University East Library, 7001 East Williams Field Road, Mesa, AZ 85212 (E-mail: bdangelo@asu.edu).

The author would like to thank Michael R. Moore, Instructor for TWC421, for his enthusiastic support and commitment to this project.

[Haworth co-indexing entry note]: "If They Build It Will They Come? Cooperation and Collaboration to Create a Customized Library." D'Angelo, Barbara J. Co-published simultaneously in *The Reference Librarian* (The Haworth Information Press, an imprint of The Haworth Press, Inc.) No. 83/84, 2003, pp. 237-250; and: *Cooperative Reference: Social Interaction in the Workplace* (ed: Celia Hales Mabry) The Haworth Information Press, an imprint of The Haworth Press, Inc., 2003, pp. 237-250. Single or multiple copies of this article are available for a fee from The Haworth Document Delivery Service [1-800-HAWORTH, 9:00 a.m. - 5:00 p.m. (EST). E-mail address: docdelivery@haworthpress.com].

Digital Object Identifier: 10.1300J120v40n83_19

orating to integrate coursework and activities into the new MWTC on-line degree curriculum to prepare students to take a proactive and decision-making role in information resource and service selection, organization, and system design. The resulting product will be a truly user-centered designed library portal and an educational methodology which may be used for the design of portals for other campus programs. *[Article copies available for a fee from The Haworth Document Delivery Service: 1-800-HAWORTH. E-mail address: <docdelivery@haworthpress.com> Website: <http://www.HaworthPress.com> © 2003 by The Haworth Press, Inc. All rights reserved.]*

KEYWORDS. Portal, faculty-library collaboration, community

INTRODUCTION

Arizona State University (ASU) East, located in the rapidly growing East Valley area of Phoenix, is one of the campuses of the tri-campus ASU system. Founded in 1996, ASU East offers unique degree programs and has a current student population of approximately 3,200 with anticipated growth to 5,000 students by 2005. One of the hallmarks of ASU East as a campus is its strong commitment to community, both the academic community on campus and the larger community in which the campus is located. For example, one of the ASU East librarians led the establishment of a Boys and Girls Club on campus to serve the day care needs of families living on campus as well as the childcare needs of commuting faculty, students, and staff. She remains instrumental in the success of the Club and has received several grant awards to fund its reading program.

ASU East Library is a "hybrid library" consisting of a predominantly electronic collection. The library maintains a small book and print periodical collection representing core materials related to campus programs. Access to a broader range of print resources is available at no cost to ASU East-affiliated patrons through electronic document delivery from the collections of ASU Tempe, ASU West in Phoenix, and commercial vendors. The document delivery service provides students with a far greater range of research materials than are available locally in print or through full-text databases and eliminates the need to travel to other campuses or other libraries to conduct additional research. Although not the traditional model for an academic library, East Library represents the transformational nature of contemporary libraries from physical to electronic access. In line with this delivery of information and service in the electronic environment, East Library has developed a number of services available through the Web including forms to request services, a searchable index of Internet resources related to ASU East programs, and a Voice-over-IP reference service piloted in Spring 2003. ASU East Librarians have created Quickstart Guides (subject-specific research guides) for various discipline areas, providing links to relevant research resources and assistance. At the same time, East Library has a strong commitment to personalized service. Reference and research assistance are available from East librarians in person, by phone, through e-mail, and beginning January 2003 remotely via Voice-over-IP. Librarians also conduct instruction sessions for individual classes and collaborate with faculty on the design of library assignments for their classes and programs. In addition, two 3-credit classes, "InfoGlut: Deal With It," and "Information Architecture" are taught by a librarian under the umbrella of the Multimedia Writing and Technical Communication Program.

The Multimedia Writing and Technical Communication Program (MWTC) focuses on the production, design, and management of information using both traditional and leading edge technologies. Students learn to communicate, both orally and in writing, across audiences and cultures; issues of ethics in technical communication; to be aware of the global nature of technical communication–both culturally and economically; to evaluate print, oral, and electronic sources; to understand appropriate technical genres; to incorporate appropriate visual elements and design in written documents and oral presentations; and to work in appropriate media. One of the purposes of the Program is to strengthen students' skills and to give them as much experience as possible in environments which approximate the workplace. These objectives make the MWTC Program an ideal collaborator for the Library and this project.

LITERATURE REVIEW

According to the *Oxford English Dictionary* two definitions of "community" include "social intercourse; fellowship, communion" and "life in association with others; society, the social state" (Oxford, 1971). Within a university setting there are many instances of communities of fellowship and society. Academic programs and departments are communities of interest formed among faculty and students that exist within the broader community of an individual college which in turn exists within the broader community of the university. Individuals may also belong to additional communities of interest both internal and external to the university environment such as student groups, professional societies or associations, and personal interest groups. Communities have been a component of the electronic environment since the beginning of the Internet. Going under many names (community networks, community information systems, online communities, web communities, etc.), virtual communities use various technologies to extend the concept of community to the online environment by encouraging, facilitating, and promoting social interaction among those with common interests. Indeed, the nature of the technology allows for communities to be extended beyond the physical limits of geographic boundaries. Virtual communities have existed since the inception of the Internet and prior to the development of the World Wide Web. Several innovative faculty early on recognized and developed their potential for teaching and learning and more recently they have received increased attention as an instructional tool. For example, virtual communities were a National Learning Infrastructure Initiative key theme for 2002 in recognition of the social interaction that is necessary for learning and the construction of knowledge (National Learning Infrastructure Initiative, 2002).

In *The 12 Principles of Civilization*, Mongoose Technology outlines twelve principles of collaboration essential for communities of any type (Mongoose, 2001):

- Purpose (Community exists because the members share a common purpose which can only be accomplished jointly.)
- Identity (Members can identify each other and build relationships.)
- Reputation (Members build a reputation based on the expressed opinions of others.)
- Governance (The facilitators and members of the community assign management duties to each other, allowing the community to grow.)
- Communication (Members must be able to interact with each other.)
- Groups (Community members group themselves according to specific interests or tasks.)
- Environment (A synergistic environment enables community members to achieve their purpose.)
- Boundaries (The community knows why it exists and what or who is outside and inside.)
- Trust (Building trust between members and with community facilitators increases group efficiency and enables conflict resolution.)

- Exchange (The community recognizes forms of exchange values, such as knowledge, experience, support, barter or money.)
- Expression (The community itself has a 'soul' or 'personality'; members are aware of what other community members are doing.)
- History (The community must keep track of past events and must react and change in response to it.)

Adapted from Mongoose Technologies.

Although these serve as guiding principles for the design of Mongoose's software, they also serve as tenets for the development of the technologies, processes, and systems that facilitate the formation and maintenance of a collaborative virtual community. Key to virtual communities is the ability to communicate and share information. As noted by Pettigrew et al. (2002) "... the Internet has facilitated the creation of information communities–an emerging concept that describes constituencies united by a common interest in building and increasing access to a set of dynamic, linked, and varying information resources."

Libraries have taken advantage of the opportunity provided by virtual communities to forge links with local government, businesses, organizations, and service providers as well as to enhance their role as information providers. Notable among these efforts are the public library-supported community information networks evaluated by Pettigrew et al. (2002) (Three Rivers Free-Net, NorthStarNet, and CascadeLink) and Prairienet, developed and supported by the Graduate School of Library and Information Sciences at the University of Illinois, Urbana-Champaign (Prairienet, n.d.). Public libraries are a natural partner in these efforts due to their expertise in information management, their role in dissemination of community information, and their strong public service commitments.

Academic libraries, too, have a significant place within their institutions and as facilitators of community among faculty, students, and staff. Communication technologies have afforded librarians and faculty new opportunities to develop and enhance collaborative work. The creation of information communities adds a valuable new arena in which libraries may partner with others in the university setting.

As a relatively new campus, the partnerships and collaborations at ASU East are evolving both among campus departments and between the campus and external agencies. Early on the Library became involved with campus-community service ties and has sought to develop and enhance ties and partnerships with academic programs as they have become established. Shared goals of information management provide the Library and the MWTC Program with a natural foundation for collaboration. The Program's curriculum in writing and multimedia combine with an interest in technology that facilitates an interest in creative new projects such as the development of an online information system. In addition, as a young program still developing an identity, this project encourages student involvement and active participation in community building among themselves and program faculty that will also benefit future students by introducing them to the Program and discipline.

PROJECT BACKGROUND

Many libraries have developed customizable user interfaces or portals to allow patrons to create their own library gateway of relevant resources and services. These portals, frequently known as "MyLibrary," attempt to deal with the glut of information available and offer patrons the opportunity to customize their own library web page in order to overcome the sense of information overload (Morgan, 2000). For the most part, these portals permit patrons to create their library page by selecting from predefined menus that have been developed by librarians. Although patrons have the ability to customize resources and, in some cases the interface itself, their participation has been for the most part reactive in nature. For example, in the typical MyLibrary system patrons have limited, if any, ability to contribute content and communication is limited.

The MyLibrary portals currently in use mostly are designed to be customized for individual needs and use. Since MyLibrary systems have a very specific objective and goal–to overcome information overload–at first glance it would appear that the customization and personalization prevalent would be in conflict with the idea of community, particularly if customization is focused on the individual level. Much still needs to be done on the assessment of the effectiveness of MyLibrary systems; however, in one case it has been found that they work best when focused and developed for a particular course (Ghaphery, 2000). While this may be seen as an extension of the traditional course page, the technologies which make MyLibrary possible have the potential to extend and expand upon the course or subject page concept to the broader concept of online information community. The MWTC portal is intended to bridge the gap between individualized needs and Program identity and community by providing students the opportunity to develop a prototype information system as part of their coursework.

INITIATING AND DEVELOPING THE PROJECT

In a discussion with the head of the MWTC program, one of the reference and instruction librarians proposed a project in which students would develop an online information system for the Program as part of their coursework as an applied project. The goal of the project is to develop a Program library that involves students proactively in the design, development, creation, and implementation process. The Program Head was excited and felt this was a good collaborative project for the Program and the Library and that as an applied project students would gain real-world experience working with information management and design. In addition, the project capitalizes on the University's emphasis on learner-centered education through "exploration of meaning and content knowledge through personal and interpersonal discovery. The process implies active involvement by the student and the integration of academics with the student's total development" (Arizona, n.d.).

Shortly after discussing the project, the Program Head applied for an Access and Workforce Development Grant from the Arizona Board of Regents for funding to develop online classes for the Program. The collaborative portal project was included in the proposal, which was funded for courses for the 2002-03 academic year.

With word that the grant had been funded, the Program Head went ahead with plans to hire two instructors, both of whom had experience developing and teaching classes with technology. Both, however, were not part of the ASU system and one was from outside the state. In early summer, introductions were made by e-mail so that the librarian and two instructors could exchange information about the project. Although both had been briefed on the project by the Program Head, this exchange of information directly between the librarian and instructors allowed for clarification of goals and desired outcomes. During this exchange, one of the instructors determined that the project was not a good fit for the course she was developing and dropped out. The other instructor was more than interested in building the project into his class, expressing excitement at not only the potential for the project to fulfill the educational goals of the course but also to provide the students with real world experience for their portfolio that would enhance their employability upon graduation.

Over the summer the librarian and instructor began discussions to develop the class. Through at times lengthy e-mail exchanges, the two worked out details on how the class would be conducted and the library project integrated into the course content. ASU supports BlackBoard, a course management system, for distance learning and online courses. Although it would be used for this course, the instructor also decided to use a MOO (multi-media environment, object oriented) for real-time class sessions. For development of the customized library system, we decided to use the *MyLibrary@NCState* software. This open source program, originally developed at North Carolina State University by Eric Lease Morgan (now at Notre Dame University), was ideal for the project. MyLibrary "supports a framework for libraries to provide enhanced access to local and remote sets of data, information, and knowledge. At the same time, it does not overwhelm its users with too much information because the users control exactly how much information is displayed to them at any given time. The system is active and not passive; direct human interaction, computer mediated guidance and communication technologies, as well as current awareness services all play indispensable roles in its implementation" (Morgan, 2000). By beginning with an established software program such as MyLibrary, with user and administrative functions already designed, the need to create a system from scratch was eliminated so that students could concentrate on interface design, content selection, and evaluation and analysis.

As fall semester approached course design became more prominent as the instructor worked out issues of scheduling class sessions and integrating course content with the various technologies to be used. At the same time, the instructor and librarian began a discussion about assessing student learning outcomes. The project was intended to be of an applied nature to give students experience in project management and implementation; however, students' enhanced understanding of information, information management, and the role of libraries and technology were all considered to be key outcomes.

The librarian provided the instructor with a list of potential assessment areas that she wished to explore. Questions were built into either group discussions or into writing assignments dispersed throughout the course. The instructor also had the students keep reflection journals in which they would explore information-related topics and their preconceptions and assumptions. Ideally, the information and knowledge needed to complete the project would be built over the course of the semester and the purpose of the questions was to track student perceptions and attitudes and how they changed as they applied what they learned. Through application, it is believed that learning and understanding are transferable and long-lasting, two of the goals of information literacy and life-long learning. Although a completed customized library was hoped for by the end of the semester, the instructor and librarian were in agreement that the project itself was a way to build students' understanding and reflection upon information, knowledge, and the role of libraries as well as "the shifting, interactive interfaces between people, ideas, and information . . . " (Moore, October 2002). In addition, the instructor's objective was to have "students understand (and apply somewhere) more complex and reflective understandings of 'interactivity,' 'interfaces,' 'usability,' and compassionate writing and design" (Moore, October 2002).

GETTING THE BALL ROLLING

To approximate a real-world work environment, a client-consultant relationship was established between the students and the Library with the librarian serving as contact person. Students were divided into design teams and coordinated by a management team which was also responsible for communication with the client to determine project scope and priorities and regularly provide updates on progress through meetings, memos, and reports. This team was also responsible for funneling questions from other teams to the librarian and vice versa. Altogether, teams included (Moore, 2002):

- Project Management: to "create order out of chaos; plan logistics and timing of project work; provide consistent, enthusiastic feedback & reinforcement to all Design Teams (be strict when you have to); communicate with Project Client (Barbara D'Angelo), and with Library IT support (Pedro Carrasquilla)";
- Portal Categories and Content: responsible for " . . . appropriate, creative, meaningful categories & content for MTWC-specific Portal";
- Interface Design and Documentation: responsible for "Web-Based Portal design; layout; 'look & feel'; colors; typefaces. Documentation";
- Graphics and Audience Analysis: responsible for "Graphics–banners, images, buttons, icons, photos, etc.";
- Usability and Community Relations: responsible for " . . . at least one Paper Prototyping Session, one Usability Session, & one public ASU-EAST Presentation";
- Project Ethnographer: to "Observe & Report on Project Progress, CMC interactions; collaborative protocols & interactions."

Students were to document the project through the use of various types of writing: memos and e-mail for communication between teams and between the class and the client and reports for ensuring that all aspects of the project and procedures were documented. At the end of the semester students were to complete a final report to the client outlining progress to-date and recommendations for future development and maintenance. By mid-semester, the librarian and instructor determined that a workable prototype may not be completed by semester's end. However, since the instructor would be teaching the same course during Spring 2003, they decided that the project would carry over. This increased the importance for the students to produce clear and precise documentation since new teams would pick up on and take over their work. It also added to the "real-world" experience for the students in the sense of team member turnover.

A project timeline was developed to provide students with guidance on work that needed to be accomplished by the end of the semester. The instructor built web pages for each team to provide guidance and background information not only for the project task they were assigned but also to provide guidance in team building, role responsibilities, and project management. Some initial confusion ensued as the Project Management team worked through the details and chaos of facilitating work among the groups. Leadership emerged among the individual teams as well as for the overall project within the Project Management group while others appeared at times to be overwhelmed by the tasks assigned to them and by the amount of communication among and between groups.

In mid-October, the instructor gave the class the green light to begin working on the project. The first meeting between the Project Management team and the librarian as client took place later in the month when the team presented the client with their completed audience analysis and progress update. Meetings ensued between students and the client over the next few weeks as questions arose about technical issues with the software and confusion set in on the types of content to be used. In preparing the students to work on the project, the instructor spent class time and assigned out-of-class reading materials on project management and on professional communication and working with clients. Project Management team members were expected to approach the librarian as client, not teacher. This expectation was difficult to achieve particularly since two lead students on the Project Management team were enrolled in a course taught by the librarian, thereby already having an established teacher-student relationship. In addition, because the instructor was distant and not readily available for in-person meetings, the librarian became at times the point person for questions.

The instructor made an in-person visit in mid-November to meet students face-to-face for the first time allowing for more in-depth discussions with the various teams and resolution of any problems they were experiencing but reluctant to express in online meetings. Although students were already engaged in the project, the visit re-energized their work and allowed them to tackle some of the issues that seemed to bog them down.

BUILDING COMMUNITY

One of the results of the project has been the building of a working relationship between the instructor in the MWTC Program and the librarian. Building on similar backgrounds and philosophy for the use of technology in instruction and the importance of information, they were able to readily agree on all aspects of the course and the integration of the project into the class design. While a good relationship already existed between the Library and the MWTC Program, this project assisted in enhancing the collaboration and partnership between the two.

Another result of the project has been relationship building among the MWTC students as they worked through many of the issues involved in selecting the content and creating the structure of the portal. The class worked together to create a new name for the portal that would be more reflective of the portal concept and of their community. The Graphics and Audience Analysis team developed a new logo for the portal to replace the North Carolina-specific graphic which came with the software. Renaming the portal and creating a new logo in particular lent themselves to community building since both provided the students with the opportunity to establish an identity for their Program.

Other alterations to the design and appearance of the software created opportunities for the students to reflect on their roles as creators of Program community. They wrote an "About" page explaining the purpose of the portal and their role in its development, revised help pages to assist users in creating accounts and customizing the portal. They developed a "disciplines" page describing the various areas of study and knowledge within the MWTC Program. While creating this page, Project Management Team members expressed awareness that the discipline descriptions could be used by newly enrolled students to introduce themselves to the specialized areas within the Program.

Selecting and categorizing content also provided opportunities for community building. Students struggled somewhat with content issues for themselves and also for faculty and new incoming students. This awareness of building a portal for the long-term and for making it viable and relevant to new students enrolled in the Program was evident early on as the teams worked on their audience analysis and grappled with the need to create categories of content that would assist new students to become part of the MWTC community and also to facilitate students' progress through the Program in their particular area of interest. One area of mild conflict was over "appropriate" subject matter and whether links should be included to content other than academic and professional. Several students desired links to entertainment and communication areas in addition to the more serious content for research. This became an issue of contention for several weeks as communication broke down between the Project Management and Portal Categories and Content teams. Project Management team members approached the librarian/client several times for clarification about appropriate content and for suggestions for categories and content links. Although final decisions about content rested initially with the Project Management team, final decisions about links and categories resided with the librarian.

Although building and enhancing community within ASU East was primary, the selection and use of the MyLibrary software provided an ideal venue for contributing to community beyond the walls of ASU East. As an open source product, the MyLibrary development community is active and maintains a listserv of interested parties to follow the software's development and contribute new information about ongoing projects. The instructor wrote to Eric Lease Morgan to inform him that the class would be using the MyLibrary software for the project. Mr. Morgan's response was enthusiastic support, which he continued to voice. The librarian posted a message to the listserv in mid-October in order to introduce the ASU East project to the entire development group and to solicit feedback and comments as well as build a potential base of experts who would be able and willing to advise on the project if necessary. Unfortunately, feedback was limited. The student webmaster posted a message late in the semester inquiring about copyright issues related to the software. In addition to receiving a response, he was also encouraged to post impressions about the software and to engage in feedback about its use.

CURRENT STATUS AND FUTURE WORK

At the time of writing teams are finalizing their work, the webmaster for the project and the systems administrator are completing work on the initial design of the portal, documentation and final reports are being prepared, and a presentation is being readied for unveiling of the portal to the MWTC Program members and to the Library as a whole in mid-December. The Library will link the portal from its current website for ready access for students and faculty and also as a demo project of a user-defined customized library system.

Work will continue on content development, interface design, and usability in the spring 2003 class taught by the same instructor. The student webmaster for the project has committed to continuing for the spring semester as an internship thereby lending consistency and continuity to the project. He not only will bring project memory but also leadership as he has been instrumental to the project's success. This follow-up and continued development over multiple semesters will also aid in the development of the portal as a "community" tool for the Program and Library as it becomes ingrained within the instructional goals for the Program and as part of the students' experience as members of the MWTC community.

REFERENCES

Arizona Faculties Council "Learner-Centered Defined." (n.d.) Available at http://ag.arizona.edu/azlearners/afcdefined-learnercentered.html. Retrieved 26 June 2002.

Ghaphery, Jimmy and Dan Ream (2000), "VCU's MyLibrary: Librarians Love It. . . . Users? Well, Maybe," *Information Technology and Libraries* 19 (December), 186-190.

Mongoose Technology (2001), "The 12 Principles of Civilization." Available at http://www.mongoosetech.com/realcommunities/12prin.html. Retrieved 26 June 2002.

Moore, Michael (2 October 2002), Personal Communication.

Moore, Michael (2002), "Fall 2002 Library Portal Project Teams and Responsibilities." Available at http://twc.composing.org/portal/groups/. Retrieved 14 November 2002.

Morgan, Eric Lease (2000), "The Challenges of User-Centered, Customizable Interfaces to Library Resources," *Information Technology and Libraries* 19 (December), 166-168.

Morgan, Eric Lease (1999), "MyLibrary@NCState: The Implementation of a User-Centered, Customizable Interface to a Library's Collection of Information Resources." Available at http://dewey.library.nd.edu/mylibrary/sigir-99/. Retrieved 3 October 2002.

National Learning Infrastructure Initiative Meeting Notes 2002 (2002), Available at http://www.educause.edu/ir/library/pdf/NLI0211.pdf. Retrieved 24 October 2002.

The Compact Edition of the Oxford English Dictionary: Complete Text Reproduced Micrographically. (1971) Volume I A-O. New York: Oxford University Press, 486.

Pettigrew, Karen K., Joan C. Durrance, and Kenton T. Unruh (2002), "Facilitating Community Information Seeking Using the Internet: Findings from Three Public Library-Community Network Systems." *Journal of the American Society for Information Science and Technology* 53 (1), 894-903.

Prairienet Community Network (n.d.) Available at http://www.prairienet.org/about/. Retrieved 14 November 2002.

COOPERATING
WITH OTHER LIBRARIES

A National Laboratory
and University Branch Campus
Library Partnership:
Shared Benefits and Challenges
from Combined Reference Services

Karen A. Buxton
Harvey R. Gover

SUMMARY. The Hanford Technical Library of the Pacific Northwest National Laboratory and the Max E. Benitz Memorial Library of the Washington State University Tri-Cities Branch Campus have functioned

Karen A. Buxton is Information Specialist, Hanford Technical Library, Pacific Northwest National Laboratory, P.O. Box 999, Richland, WA 99352 (E-mail: karen.buxton@pnl.gov). Harvey R. Gover is Assistant Campus Librarian, Max E. Benitz Memorial Library, Washington State University at Tri-Cities, 2710 University Drive, Richland, WA 99352-1671 (E-mail: hgover@tricity.wsu.edu).

[Haworth co-indexing entry note]: "A National Laboratory and University Branch Campus Library Partnership: Shared Benefits and Challenges from Combined Reference Services." Buxton, Karen A., and Harvey R. Gover. Co-published simultaneously in *The Reference Librarian* (The Haworth Information Press, an imprint of The Haworth Press, Inc.) No. 83/84, 2003, pp. 251-262; and: *Cooperative Reference: Social Interaction in the Workplace* (ed: Celia Hales Mabry) The Haworth Information Press, an imprint of The Haworth Press, Inc., 2003, pp. 251-262. Single or multiple copies of this article are available for a fee from The Haworth Document Delivery Service [1-800-HAWORTH, 9:00 a.m. - 5:00 p.m. (EST). E-mail address: docdelivery@haworthpress.com].

http://www.haworthpress.com/web/REF
Digital Object Identifier: 10.1300J120v40n83_20

both separately and in combination since moving into the same space within the Consolidated Information Center in 1997. The libraries have successfully partnered to serve different clientele at a combined reference desk since June 1997. Although having separate staffs, catalogs, and collections, the libraries share a single reference/information desk. The reference staffs work together to serve a very diverse clientele including students, faculty, engineers, scientists, contractors, regulators, and the public. The combined libraries offer significant benefits to both library staffs and their users. The libraries have expanded access to collections and information expertise, enhanced staff training opportunities, and provided additional hours of reference service to patrons while at the same time maintaining the individual identities of the two libraries. *[Article copies available for a fee from The Haworth Document Delivery Service: 1-800-HAWORTH. E-mail address: <docdelivery@haworthpress.com> Website: <http://www.HaworthPress.com>* © *2003 by The Haworth Press, Inc. All rights reserved.]*

KEYWORDS. Hanford Technical Library, Pacific Northwest National Laboratory, Washington State University Tri-Cities, Max E. Benitz Memorial Library, combined reference desk, consolidated libraries, merged libraries, combined libraries, merged reference

INTRODUCTION

Libraries are discovering opportunities to improve services, enhance collections, and meet the needs of changing clientele through partnerships. The Hanford Technical Library (HTL) (2002) and the Max E. Benitz Memorial Library (Benitz Library) (2002) share space in the Consolidated Libraries, a single facility on the Washington State University (WSU) Tri-Cities (2002) branch campus, and have successfully partnered to serve different clientele at a combined reference desk since June 1997. This unusual partnership allows both libraries to provide additional hours of reference service, access to greater library resources for each clientele, and facilitates access to the Consolidated Libraries, an important regional information resource for citizens of the Tri-Cities of Richland, Kennewick, and Pasco and the surrounding Columbia Basin region of southeastern Washington State. Searching the literature reveals that partnerships in which different types of libraries share building space are not entirely unknown but remain uncommon. This partnership of a medium-sized, federally funded technical library and a relatively small university branch-campus library provides great benefit to clients and the community, and at the same time, presents some management and human relations challenges.

The Consolidated Libraries (2002) are a unit within the Consolidated Information Center (CIC) (2002). The CIC is located on the WSU Tri-Cities branch campus by the Columbia River in north Richland, seven to ten miles from Kennewick and Pasco, and on the southern boundary of the U.S. Department of Energy (DOE) Hanford Site (2002), formerly the Hanford Nuclear Reservation. The Consolidated Libraries also house the DOE Public Reading Room (2002) and the Southeastern Washington Business Information Center (BIC), a local business extension program (Business LINKS, 2002).

While the DOE Reading Room and BIC have separate quarters and operations within the Consolidated Libraries, the HTL and the Benitz Library combine portions of their collections and some of their public services operations. For example, the two libraries have integrated their physical circulating and reference book collections and the paper journal collections into single arrangements. The circulation and reference desks are likewise integrated and staffed by both libraries. The two libraries, however, have separate administrations; separate funding sources and staffs; and separate online information resources, catalogs, and circulation systems.

DESCRIPTION OF THE LIBRARIES

Hanford Technical Library

The HTL is a unit of the Pacific Northwest National Laboratory (PNNL) (2002), a DOE multi-program national laboratory. PNNL is operated under contract on behalf of DOE by the Pacific Northwest Division of the Battelle Memorial Institute, a non-profit science and technology research organization based in Columbus, Ohio (Battelle, 2002). The HTL serves about 12,700 employees of PNNL, Hanford Site contractors, local DOE personnel, as well as serving local and regional companies and agencies that contract for library services. These constituent groups are spread over the 586 square miles of the Hanford Site (U.S. Department of Energy-Richland Operations Office, 2002); the cities of Richland, Kennewick, and Pasco; and regionally within Washington and Oregon. The primary objective of the HTL is to support the science and technology research of PNNL, the clean-up operations of Hanford Site contractors, and the legal and regulatory functions of DOE. The HTL has a staff of 24.2 full-time equivalent (FTE) employees. The collections have a science and technology focus and include 38,000 books, approximately 1,100 current journals, 90,000 bound journal volumes, and over 800,000 technical reports published at PNNL, other national laboratories, and by other government organizations.

The Benitz Library

The Benitz Library is one of three branch campus libraries in the WSU System (Washington State University, 2002). The Benitz Library serves the approximately 1,300 students who take classes at the Richland campus and at the Yakima and Wenatchee Learning Centers, each more than two hours driving time away. The Benitz Library also serves over 50 full-time faculty and a pool of more than 350 adjunct faculty drawn from the surrounding communities, PNNL, and the Hanford "brain trust" of highly qualified scientists and professionals (Washington State University Tri-Cities, 2002), many of whom are also HTL clients.

The Benitz Library staffing level is 6.2 FTE and it holds an on-site collection of 20,000 books, 176 journal subscriptions, and 758,116 research documents and ERIC microfiche.

The Benitz Library collections support degree programs in agriculture; electrical, environmental, and mechanical engineering; computer science; business; education; biology; chemistry; nursing; and liberal arts.

HISTORY OF THE COMBINED LIBRARIES

The HTL and Benitz Library share parallel histories of service to the Hanford Site beginning shortly after plutonium production was underway in 1945. The WSU Tri-Cities campus traces its origins back to the General Electric School of Nuclear Engineering, founded in 1946 to provide training for Hanford personnel (Washington State University Student Alumni Connection, 2002). The library that served the school was at that time a branch of the Hanford Site library. The name of the school and the institutions with which it has been affiliated changed over the years. Since the 1960s, several institutions jointly operated the school until it became a branch campus and the exclusive responsibility of WSU in 1989.

The idea of merging the HTL with the WSU Tri-Cities branch campus library was first presented by PNNL in the mid-1980s. The idea grew into a proposed Consolidated Information Center (CIC) that was to include the DOE Reading Room. WSU Tri-Cities founding Dean, Dr. James Cochran, championed the proposal with WSU and the Washington State Legislature. Construction began on the CIC in December 1995.

While the building was under construction, preparations were made to create a new type of library. A detailed planning process was funded by PNNL to smooth the transition from individual organizations into one consolidated library. Initially, the idea of combining libraries was a cause for concern by some staff at both libraries. During the nineteen-month planning process and even after the move, conflict existed between the HTL and Benitz Library cultures. Despite an overlap in patron groups, HTL staff primarily serve scientific and technical professionals and Benitz Library staff serve undergraduate and graduate academic patrons. Benitz Library focuses on teaching patrons one-on-one to do their own searching and provides self-service photocopying while HTL emphasizes fee-based searching and photocopy services, and group instruction. Benitz Library patrons are primarily walk-in users while HTL provides reference services principally electronically and by phone. No guidelines existed to help the staffs blend their distinct cultures into a new combined library model (Conaway, 2000). The planning process worked out the roles and responsibilities of each organization including service levels and customer support. The preparation of a staff handbook before the move to the new facility helped establish routines and clear lines of demarcation. In addition, numerous cross-training activities were set up with the goal of providing appropriate training to all employees. In June 1997, the CIC opened its doors to the people of the Mid-Columbia region to "not only provide easier access to a vast library collection, but also as a catalyst to boost the local economy" (Consolidated Information Center, 2002).

HOW THE COLLABORATION WORKS

Reference desk staffing follows the needs of the primary clientele of each library. Classes at the branch campus are held throughout the day, six days a week. Most classes, however, meet in the afternoon and evenings Monday through Thursday. PNNL and Hanford Site staffs primarily require library services Monday through Friday between 8:00 a.m. and 5:00 p.m. For these reasons, HTL staff has assumed primary responsibility for reference desk coverage weekdays during business hours, and Benitz Library employees have primary responsibility for evening and weekend coverage.

Generally two employees, one from each library, staff the reference desk Monday through Wednesday during business hours. This overlap enables HTL and Benitz Library employees to schedule and attend meetings and training sessions while assuring that reference service is available to patrons. Benitz Library staff is also able to accomplish tasks that take them away from the reference desk such as training new student employees and helping out in other areas of the library when needed. When reference staffs from both libraries are on duty their patrons are divided respectively. However, during shifts when only one reference specialist is on duty, that individual serves all patrons and helps anyone who requests assistance at the combined reference desk. New users of the Consolidated Libraries are often unaware that multiple libraries are operating out of the same space.

The HTL library staff provides basic reference service at no charge to its client groups. However, in-depth reference questions, literature searches, and other information services requiring thirty minutes or more to complete are charged back to the client's research account. For this reason, HTL librarians provide only basic reference services to patrons other than their own who come to the desk for help. Whenever possible, Benitz Library reference personnel are called to the desk to handle in-depth reference questions from their patrons, during shifts when there is not already a Benitz Library staff member on duty. On occasions when in-depth reference service is needed and no Benitz Library staff is available, contact information is provided so that patrons can set up an appointment with a librarian.

The Consolidated Libraries share a commitment to providing remote electronic access to information for their respective patrons. HTL patrons are spread over a large geographical area and coming to the library is inconvenient and often impractical. HTL provides online resources to its main customer groups via the PNNL Intranet and Hanford local area network, extending many library services to patrons' desktops. Books and library materials are available to eligible users through *Leona*, the HTL online catalog. In addition PNNL and Hanford site employees may checkout and renew library materials online via *Leona*. Access to online indexes and full-text services outside Leona is similarly provided from the HTL Intranet pages. Similarly, *Griffin*, the online catalog of the WSU System, provides remote access to a wide range of electronic information services via the Web to all WSU users having an active WSU identification number. The Benitz Library functions primarily as a gateway to the much more extensive collections of the WSU libraries and offers academic patrons at the branch campus many more resources than the Benitz Library could otherwise provide. The collections available through *Griffin* are extended through *Cascade*, the online union catalog from all the other Washington State-supported institutions of higher learning (Max E. Benitz Memorial Library, 2002). *Griffin* users may expand searches directly into *Cascade*, and those with active WSU identification numbers may request that books be sent to them in both *Griffin* and *Cascade*. The libraries offer two rows of user stations with easy access to the reference desk. One row is set up to access the WSU gateway and the other row is configured for HTL online resources. All reference staff members are expected to be familiar with the electronic resources that both libraries provide.

The reference staffs are cross-trained and equipped to handle most general questions presented by the counterpart's library patrons. Occasionally, questions must be referred, and these situations initiate much of the informal training that takes place between Benitz Library and HTL staffs. Cross-training usually involves one-on-one instruction between employees. HTL staff must be able to help WSU students and faculty use databases, locate research materials, and answer a variety of policy questions. WSU staff is asked about accessing the closed stacks in the HTL Technical Reports area, locating industry codes and standards, and finding materials on a variety of technical and scientific topics. In addition, electronic resources on both sides of the aisle are updated as interfaces change. The overlapping reference desk coverage allows both staffs to get timely answers to institution-specific questions. This informal training leads to a better understanding of our counterpart's tools and processes and results in better service to patrons.

As noted earlier, the DOE Reading Room and BIC maintain separate operations and offer services from other locations within the Consolidated Libraries. Reference desk personnel often meet patrons of these service areas first and then refer them to the appropriate offices. In addition, reference services are available from a separate desk at the legal branch of the HTL, located in the Federal Building in downtown Richland. These staff members have special expertise and offer important consulting relationships to the joint reference desk staff and their patrons. For example, the DOE Reading Room's browsing collection of

Hanford reports and documents and the staff knowledge regarding Hanford Site history resources is a boon to many researchers. Legal Library branch employees are just a telephone call away. They are always willing to offer help in identifying and locating laws, statutes, and other legal information. These experts extend the ability of joint reference desk staff to provide excellent service to patrons. At the same time, DOE Reading Room and Legal Library staffs refer patron questions back to the joint reference desk when appropriate.

PARTNERSHIP BENEFITS

Patrons of the HTL and Benitz libraries benefit from the reference desk collaboration. Before the consolidation, the Benitz Library did not provide reference desk staffing during all hours it was open, and the HTL provided reference assistance only during business hours. Cooperation between the two organizations now permits reference desk coverage every hour that the libraries are open, thereby providing all patrons with increased services.

Each library has sponsored a variety of training classes and has offered participation to partner library staff. The WSU library has access to a computer lab for hands-on Web and computer database training. The collaboration provides greater access to training for both staffs.

The physical collections of each library have been selected to serve the needs of its own clientele, yet the subject emphases complement each other. Both collections are cataloged according to the Library of Congress classification and are easy to browse on the shelves. Patrons from PNNL, the Hanford Site, students, staff, and faculty all benefit from access to the combined collections, because they have circulation privileges at both libraries. The strength of the HTL scientific and technical collections are of particular use to post-graduate students at WSU, while the Benitz Library and BIC business collections augment HTL resources. In addition, walk-in users have access to the electronic journals and databases of both libraries, many of which are unique to one library or the other.

The HTL and Benitz Library also coordinate selection of materials for collection development. The Benitz Library was able to cancel some subscriptions and standing orders for materials the HTL also purchased. Each library was also able to provide new focus to its collection development budget. The Benitz Library was able to concentrate spending on business, social sciences, the humanities, and education, while the HTL continued to focus collection development dollars for science and technology purchases. Each library benefits from informal cooperative collection development activities.

PNNL proposed the partnership in the 1980s, because of its commitment to being a community and regional resource. The consolidation contributes to that strategic goal. Before moving into the CIC building, the HTL was less visible as a community resource, even though it was open to the public. The CIC offers an attractive, publicly accessible building to house the collections and resources of the participating libraries.

PARTNERSHIP CHALLENGES

The combined libraries offer significant benefits to both the HTL and Benitz Library staffs and to their respective clientele. The libraries have expanded access to collections and to information expertise, enhanced staff training opportunities, and provided additional hours of reference service to customers. The consolidation appears to provide clear advantages; however, it has also experienced some important challenges. The libraries have different missions, parent organizations, cultures, and follow different processes. All of these differences create an environment in which misunderstandings can flourish. As Dunn and Grealy observed about another academic and special library collaboration, "It took time, effort, and personal commitment on the part of all staff involved to marry two very different libraries" (Dunn and Grealy, 1996). We certainly found this to be true and believe that the effort is ongoing. As in any successful relationship, the participants must continually nurture good communications, be flexible and cooperative, and address the needs of each organization as well as those of the joint operation.

The Consolidated Libraries serve a broad-based, combined clientele. In addition to serving the information needs of PNNL, Hanford Site contractors, and the staff, faculty, and students at the WSU branch campus, the facility is open to the public. Reference staffs respond to questions from teachers, high school students, students from other colleges, small business owners, and the general public. The libraries provide different levels of service to each of these groups. For example, it is confusing to the public to discover that Benitz Library staff is unlimited in the amount of time they are able to spend providing reference assistance, while HTL limits the amount of assistance provided to each walk-in patron. Although this issue arises infrequently, it creates a public relations challenge for both staffs. Understanding and explaining policies and client services to users is an important yet difficult aspect of providing service at the combined reference desk. The book collections are integrated, but the online catalogs are not. Users must check both the HTL and WSU catalogs to find what is available in their combined collections. Much training is required to help patrons find materials. The emphasis on desktop delivery of electronic resources by both libraries presents yet another challenge. Resources available to HTL patrons via the PNNL Intranet are not available to Benitz Library staff and their patrons at their desktops. In addition, most resources available from the WSU Gateway are not available on the desktop of HTL staff. This hampers the ability of both staffs to provide customers with telephone reference. Initially, joint licensing agreements for electronic resources were considered, so that the two libraries could offer some of the same resources to all clients. The complications of negotiating license agreements for a corporate and academic library coupled with contrasting copyright restrictions and the technical challenges of operating online resources over multiple networks derailed these efforts. Changes in licensing requirements may provide future opportunities to acquire joint licensing agreements.

Communication between the staffs of the two libraries may be the greatest challenge. The directors of the two organizations strive to keep both staffs informed of changes that will affect them. Sometimes the directors do not foresee that a change at one organization will have an impact on the employees of the other. Much of the information exchange has been informal, through direct staff interaction. Although this is a great way to learn skills and transfer knowledge, it doesn't fully ensure that everyone who needs relevant information and training gets it. Recent efforts to provide new and more formal methods of information sharing promise to improve communication among staff members. For example, the directors of both libraries recently scheduled formal joint management meetings, and the heads of reference for the libraries are discussing reviving joint reference meetings to offer a venue for formal and ongoing cross-training and discussion.

THE PATH FORWARD

Paul Wasserman says "connections"–not "collections"–will become the unique challenge for providers of information services in the future

(InfoThink, 2002). Joint programs are one way to reinforce the connections among the Consolidated Libraries and draw their research missions more closely together. Recently, the parent institutions of each library, PNNL, and WSU Tri-Cities jointly hired a scientist to design a post-graduate molecular biosciences program (Maloof, 2002). This program and other joint research projects in agricultural products and "bio-based" fuels remind us that the libraries' parent institutions are connected and that they share many of the same research goals. Leveraging these connections will provide the libraries with unique opportunities to serve the researchers and institutions they support. The successful path forward lies in building on the strengths of the partnership, surmounting the impediments to providing excellent reference service, and exploring new ways to jointly serve our clientele.

REFERENCES

Battelle. Working with Battelle. Contracting with the Pacific Northwest Division of Battelle Memorial Institute. Battelle Memorial Institute Web Site. Accessed 11-17-2002. Available from http://www.battelle.org/workingwithbattelle/pnl.stm.
Business LINKS, Southeastern Washington Business Information Center. "What is the Southeastern Washington Business Information Center at Business LINKS?" Accessed 11-17-2002. Available from http://www.tricity.wsu.edu/links/bic.htm.
Conaway, Peggy. "One Reference Service for Everyone? Designing the Service for a Combined Public/Academic Library." *Library Journal.* 125[12], 42-44. 2000.
Consolidated Information Center. Washington State University Tri-Cities. Accessed 11-17-2002. Available from http://www.tricity.wsu.edu/ConsolidatedInformation Center.html.
Consolidated Libraries. Washington State University Tri-Cities Web Site Accessed 10-10-2002. Available from http://www.tricity.wsu.edu/dis/consolid.htm.
Dunn, Lisa G. and Deborah S. Grealy. "The Industry Information Center Within an Academic Library. A Case Study. Natural Gas Supply Information Center at Colorado School of Mines, 1985-1995." *Special Libraries* 87 [Summer], 169-80. 1996.
Hanford Technical Library. Pacific Northwest National Laboratory. Accessed 12-01-2002. Available from http://www.pnl.gov/tech_lib/home.html.
InfoThink: Practical Strategies for Using Information in Business. Profiles. Accessed 11-14-2002. Available from http://www.informationconsultancy.com/infothnp.htm.
Maloof, Staci. "WSU, PNNL Join in Building Biosciences Programs." PNNL Press Release, 2-28-2002, Accessed 11-21-2002. Available from http://www.pnl.gov/news/2002/02-03.htm.
Max E. Benitz Memorial Library. Accessed 11-27-2002. Available from http://www.tricity.wsu.edu/dis/maxben.htm.
Pacific Northwest National Laboratory. Accessed 12-01-2002. Available from http://www.pnl.gov.

U.S. Department of Energy Hanford Site. Accessed 12-01-2002. Available from http://www.hanford.gov/.

U.S. Department of Energy. Richland Operations Office. Accessed 11-17-2002. Available from http://www.hanford.gov/rl/siteinfo/knowus.asp.

U.S. Department of Energy Public Reading Room. Richland Operations Office. Office of River Protection. Accessed 12-01-2002. Available from http://reading-room.pnl.gov/.

Washington State University Student Alumni Connection. WSU Heritage/History. Accessed 11-18-2002. Available from http://www.wsu.edu/~sac/heritage/history/1940.htm.

Washington State University Tri-Cities. Accessed 12-01-2002. Available from http://www2.tricity.wsu.edu/.

When the Walls Came Tumbling Down: The Development of Cooperative Service and Resource Sharing in Libraries: 1876-2002

Joseph E. Straw

SUMMARY. This article will look at the historical development of cooperative service and resource sharing in libraries. Interlibrary Loan, union catalogs, library consortia, and electronic reference, have all impacted library work in the past century. The dissolving of walls is one of the main themes of library history in the 20th century. The developments of these years has clearly put the ability to use both human and institutional resources at the heart of contemporary library service. In looking at how this came to be, this article will examine developments in societal infrastructure and technology that made cooperative schemes both possible and economical. This article will also discuss how these developments have forced libraries to consider cooperative ways to respond to their primary service function. Lastly, conclusions will be drawn about how the emerging cooperative environment is changing the educational role of the librarian. *[Article copies available for a fee from The Haworth Document Delivery Service: 1-800-HAWORTH. E-mail address: <docdelivery@haworthpress.com> Website: <http://www.HaworthPress.com> © 2003 by The Haworth Press, Inc. All rights reserved.]*

Joseph E. Straw is Associate Professor of Library Administration, University of Illinois at Urbana-Champaign, Reference Library, Room 300, Main Library, 1408 West Gregory Drive, Urbana, IL 61801 (E-mail: jstraw@uiuc.edu).

[Haworth co-indexing entry note]: "When the Walls Came Tumbling Down: The Development of Cooperative Service and Resource Sharing in Libraries: 1876-2002." Straw, Joseph E. Co-published simultaneously in *The Reference Librarian* (The Haworth Information Press, an imprint of The Haworth Press, Inc.) No. 83/84, 2003, pp. 263-276; and: *Cooperative Reference: Social Interaction in the Workplace* (ed: Celia Hales Mabry) The Haworth Information Press, an imprint of The Haworth Press, Inc., 2003, pp. 263-276. Single or multiple copies of this article are available for a fee from The Haworth Document Delivery Service [1-800-HAWORTH, 9:00 a.m. - 5:00 p.m. (EST). E-mail address: docdelivery@haworthpress.com].

Digital Object Identifer: 10.1300J120v40n83_21

KEYWORDS. Library cooperation, library history, library consortia, electronic reference

INTRODUCTION

For more than a century rapid change and technical innovation has been part of the history of libraries. Central to these historical changes has been the ability to access and use resources that exist outside the walls of any particular library. The developments of these years have clearly put cooperative use of both human and institutional resources at the heart of contemporary library service. This article will examine how resource sharing and cooperation between libraries became possible, and how developments in technology and societal infrastructure made such changes desirable. Benchmark periods will be identified and innovations like interlibrary loan, union catalogs, library consortia, and electronic reference will be highlighted as examples of cooperative frameworks that have impacted the work that librarians do everyday.

COOPERATION ON THE HORIZON: 1876-1900

The essence of cooperative library work is the ability to access resources, services, and expertise, from other places. Early library pioneers in America envisioned the need for libraries to work together in trying to provide basic resources. Samuel S. Green, the head of the Worchester Free Public Library wrote in 1876: "It would add greatly to the usefulness of our reference libraries if an agreement should be made to lend books to each other for short periods of time" (Green, 1876). In that same year, at the first conference of the American Library Association, a Cooperation Committee was set up with the charge of encouraging cooperative efforts between libraries. Some of the early questions this committee wrestled with were interlibrary lending, uniform catalog cards, and a central borrowing library. It was clear very early that the provision of service could be enhanced by the interlibrary exchange of resources (Kraus, 1975).

Despite strong intellectual support among leaders of the library profession, actual library cooperation was slow in developing. The realities of library institutions in the second half of the 19th century mitigated against cooperative efforts. The practical problems of distance were still considerable making library exchanges both time consuming and expensive. Many library institutions were just getting off the ground, and naturally they put their resources into building and classifying local collections. The ideals of modern library service were also in their infancy, with older restrictive and custodial ideals providing strong resistance to cooperative ventures. It is not surprising to find that early cooperative visions were proposed before they could be practically implemented (Stuart, 1975).

Most of the cooperative work in these years was local and on a small scale. Limited interlibrary borrowing and some shared cataloging were successfully tried among a few large institutions. Print bibliographic tools were also applied to the problem of identifying resources that might exist outside local libraries. The emergence of union lists and individual library finding guides helped to establish a bibliographic foundation for users to access collections beyond the holdings of their particular library. In the last three decades of the 19th century, twenty-five union lists were published and these began to appear in library collections across the United States (Kraus, 1975). In 1890 Lodilla Ambrose, of Northwestern University, testifies to the use of these resources by saying:

> I keep within reach of all students a full set of the Finding-lists of the Chicago Public Library. I often refer then to these when they have exhausted the material to be found here. I have more than once gone with some of them to learn how to get what they wanted there; or have given some direction here regarding that library. (Ambrose, 1890)

The popularity of union lists led many to advocate for their continued use and expansion. Josephus Nelson Larned argued in 1897 of the need for all libraries to publish indexes and bibliographic guides to their holdings. These finding lists could be widely distributed to help library users find resources that might exist anywhere in the world (Larned, 1897).

During most of the last decades of the 19th century, enthusiasm for library cooperation was often ahead of the reality. Cooperative ventures in these years only served a small group of users and library institutions. Despite the limited scale, alternatives to local library resources had been established by 1900. Luckily, a series of developments were occurring that would greatly expand the dimension of library cooperation.

FOUNDATIONS OF COOPERATIVE LIBRARY SERVICE: 1900-1930

Interlibrary Loan

At the turn of the 20th century interlibrary loan (ILL) became the focal point of cooperation among American libraries. Frequent and reliable ILL service represents the first successful cooperative effort to impact users and libraries on a mass scale. The availability of expanded ILL options allowed libraries to tap into more and more distant collections. This extended hand helped sharpen the focus in libraries on providing for users more and varied options for getting information.

Library cooperation is closely tied to communications and their development. ILL services benefited from the consolidation of national transportation and communications networks in the last decades of the 19th and first years of the 20th century. The emergence and integration of these networks opened up the possibilities for enhanced borrowing between libraries. Reliable and efficient infrastructures did much in allowing libraries to establish regular habits of interlibrary resource sharing.

The linking of the country by rail did much to open up the doors of libraries. The expansion of rail services to areas beyond main lines was a significant feature of railway development in the first years of the 20th century. Small towns and isolated regions could now reap the benefits of having access to railroads. A railroad presence to more places allowed smaller libraries to think about tapping into the resources of libraries in the larger cities. In the early 20th century, a library promise to lend an item to another library could be backed up by a railway system that could safely ship the item and predict its arrival by a regular and reliable timetable (Stover, 1997).

Telephones were impacting large numbers of people in the early decades of the 20th century. By 1910 half the residents of some urban areas had telephone service. Libraries could use phones to contact each other directly to verify materials that might potentially be borrowed. Telephone calls could also be used to instruct users about available resources, and to set up possible borrowing transactions. Borrowing libraries with a telephone could be freed from reliance on print union lists and extended written correspondence (Fischer, 1992).

The expansion of postal service perhaps did the most in helping to regularize ILL service. Most interlibrary transactions had to be sent out as packages. Until the second decade of the 20th century, the United

States Postal Service only delivered letters. Packages had to be shipped by private carriers like American Express and Wells Fargo. These arrangements added additional costs to libraries that wished to send out resources to users from other libraries (Fuller, 1972). The problems of costs and overhead slowed the development of ILL services, and the need for more favorable postal treatment is expressed in this 1910 editorial in *Library Journal*:

> Anything in the nature of a parcel's post is fiercely opposed by the express companies and by other allies of the railroad interest, and to a large extent by local merchants, who have an undue fear of mail order houses. Librarians and other friends of a parcel's post should be as active in favor of it as these opponents are against it, and whenever the subject is up in Congress the chairman of the Post Office Committee should hear from librarians all over the country. (*Library Journal*, 1910)

In 1913 the Post Office introduced parcel post service for senders of packages, and libraries no longer had to face the extra costs associated with private shipping companies. The parcel post system provided a reliable and cheap option for libraries offering ILL services. Prepaid and insured parcel post packages would be widely used for ILL transactions by the early 1920s. The advent of parcel post dramatically increased the traffic in ILL requests, and many institutions could look at ILL as a viable service. ILL departments proliferated in libraries around the country, and by 1930 ILL service was a regular feature in most libraries.

The development of ILL service encouraged other cooperative endeavors. Union lists were improved and expanded in these years. In the mid 1920s nearly 180 published lists were available. The Library of Congress expanded its publication and distribution of catalog cards, a project that would result in the publication of the *National Union Catalog* (NUC) years later. The release of the *Union List of Serials* in 1927 provided a definitive guide to the serial holdings of other libraries. Clearly, the foundation of bibliographic verification grew with increased borrowing between library institutions (Kraus, 1975).

Opportunities for more cooperation helped give credibility to the special library movement. The special library movement began in the early 20th century as businesses and other institutions set up libraries of specialized collections to support their missions. While recognizing the importance of having a library, many of these institutions did not want to invest in extensive resources. Special librarians would have to rely on cooperation in order to do their jobs. Charles Belden in 1921 stresses the importance of cooperative efforts between special and public librarians when he writes:

> Public and special libraries in large municipalities have exceptional opportunities to work together to their mutual advantage. Collections can be made to supplement each other, a not too technical union list of rare or unusual material on a given industry can aid in placing the result of business knowledge and experience of successful firms or institutions at the instant command of those ready to profit therefrom. (Belden, 1921)

Agreements for the exchange and borrowing of materials was common between public and special libraries in these years. Special libraries were some of the first library institutions to be built on the basis of having regular cooperative arrangements (Bierbaum, 1993).

COOPERATION AS ECONOMIC NECESSITY: 1930-1940

The economic disruption of the Great Depression was a further stimulus for cooperative efforts. Along with everything else, libraries found their budgets slashed and hard pressed to keep their institutions running. Many libraries turned to other libraries to pool scarce resources. New programs began to emerge that would go beyond just the lending of resources and would extend to sharing many formally internal functions.

A number of arrangements took root during these years to provide libraries with a forum to air common problems, share materials, provide services, and pool diminished resources. Perhaps one of the largest efforts began in 1932 with the Cooperative Cataloging Program that was formed to address the expensive problem of processing and the duplication of work. In a few years 400 U.S. and Canadian libraries had contributed cataloging records for over 60,000 titles that would be published by the Library of Congress as a union list of cataloging records (Alexander, 1999).

More commonly these arrangements took place between similar libraries located in the same geographic area. In the years 1931-1939 the Cooperating Libraries of Upper New York (CLUNY) brought together seven academic libraries that met on a regular basis to solve mutual problems. This group created a union list of periodicals and coordinated the purchasing and development of microfilm collections. Duke University and the University of North Carolina in 1931 agreed to accept responsibility for certain collecting areas and to share joint cataloging records. Another group of academic libraries in Georgia consisting of Atlanta University, Morehouse College, Spelman College, Morris Brown College, and Clark College agreed in 1933 to provide joint borrowing for their users (Alexander, 1999).

The general relief efforts of the Depression saw expanded development of union bibliographic tools. Multiple projects for new union lists and catalogs were carried out in this period and at the end of the 1930s over 700 such tools had been published. In 1940 the American Library Association sponsored a study that suggested coordination of union list projects, and it also argued for greater cooperation between libraries as a whole (Kraus, 1975).

COOPERATIVE BOOM: 1940-1970

Universities and Consortia

World War II and its aftermath proved to be important in the development of cooperative programs. While the scarcity of the Depression did much to encourage cooperation, the affluence of the post-war period contributed to programs that were bigger and more ambitious. College and academic libraries would lead the way in this new period of growth in cooperative activities.

Beginning in World War II a vast amount of money was put into higher education in the United States. In the immediate post-war period, the Cold War with the Soviet Union further intensified this investment. Much of this funding went into technical and scientific research with potential military applications. Libraries benefited greatly from this expansion, seeing new buildings popping up and increased budgets to purchase new materials. Libraries were also encouraged to set up relationships that could best take advantage of collections that could most benefit research. Ruth Patrick writes that libraries in this period "had to rely more and more on access, through reciprocal arrangements, to the specialized collections of companion libraries" (Patrick, 1972).

A number of consortia programs developed that expanded the scope of cooperation to a number of different areas. The New England Depository Library was created in 1942 to jointly address the storage and overflow problems of Boston College, Harvard University, MIT, Radcliffe College, Simmons College, and Tufts University. Starting in 1948, the

Farmington Plan successfully coordinated foreign acquisitions among 60 research libraries. The formation of the Center for Research Libraries (CRL) in 1951 created a central depository for the purchase and lending of expensive and little-used research collections. Perhaps one of the most important efforts was the Medical Library Assistance Act of 1965. This federal effort farmed out collection development, interlibrary loan, and reference service from the National Library of Medicine (NLM) to eleven regional medical libraries that included large medical schools like Harvard, the University of Washington, Wayne State, UCLA, Emory, Texas, and the University of Nebraska (Weber, 1976).

After 1960 the growth of library consortia greatly accelerated. Ruth Patrick in a 1972 study of academic library consortia identified 125 such arrangements of which 90 percent were formed after 1961 (Patrick, 1972). This vast explosion perhaps illustrates one of the most pressing information problems of this period. The post-war years saw a tremendous growth in the output of scholarly literatures. In fields like the sciences, the printed literature was growing at exponential levels. Problems associated with this information explosion were coming to a head in the 1960s. The dimensions of information were simply too large for any one institution to comprehend the whole. Patrick talks about the increasing trend towards cooperation in addressing these problems:

> Awareness of the vast and growing world of information in relation, to the holdings and resources of any single library, has fostered among librarians an acute appreciation of the interdependence of most of the nation's libraries and of the requirement for some level of cooperation. Academic libraries have proposed cooperative ventures long before the other parts of their institutions expressed any interest in such ventures, and interlibrary cooperative arrangements have often been one of the more productive areas of interinstitutional agreements. (Patrick, 1972)

Banding together was seen as an advantage in handling some of the new issues created by the vast growth in new information.

Stirrings of a New Wired World

By 1970 library cooperation was well developed and involved institutions of all types. The communications framework for this system was based on railroads, surface highways, mail, and telephones. This kind of framework kept most cooperative projects at the statewide and regional levels. The post-war years would see the first successful applications of computer processing to bibliographic problems. This technology would transform the framework of library cooperation in the coming years to include national and international exchanges of unprecedented scale.

The ability to store and retrieve information is at the heart of computer processing. Visions of an automated solution to this problem was proposed long before it could be practically implemented. Perhaps the most famous vision of an information processing machine was proposed by Vannevar Bush in 1945. Bush proposed an automated system that used light and electricity to store and retrieve documents. This "MEMEX" machine had a keyboard that could help formulate and process requests for the user. "MEMEX" would also be able to remember and customize the searching and processing activity of each user. Bush and other thinkers clearly saw that finding information of all types could be aided by machines (Bush, 1945).

The first working computers came on the scene in the late 1940s. A few tiny bibliographic files were stored on magnetic tapes and run through huge mainframe computers. Most of these efforts remained experimental until the late 1950s, when magnetic tapes would be used by the government and private sectors to create informational databases of their clienteles (Neufeld and Cornog, 1986). Machine-readable magnetic tapes would eventually be picked up by commercial indexing and abstracting services in the 1960s. They were able to create machine-readable bibliographic information for their products. The National Library of Medicine (NLM) undertook such a project in 1960 by automating the production process of its *Index Medicus* print index. The NLM used this to create the MEDLARS system which they offered to the medical community in 1964. By 1970 many other indexing and abstracting services had automated their production processes and were ready to make their services available to wider audiences (Straw, 2001).

A WORLD WITHOUT WALLS: 1970-2002

Technical Framework for Change

The early 1970s saw computer databases emerge as a major factor in libraries. Much of this was made possible by changes in the storage capabilities of computers. Early mainframe computers with magnetic tapes had very limited searching and processing functions. Clumsy and cryptic batch searching made retrieval problematic, and processing through bulky mainframe computers was often hindered by slow performance and system failures. The development of hard disc storage systems would do much to address these problems. The appearance of the IBM 3330 disc drive and the IBM 360 would improve the performance of mainframe computers. These new systems would allow for the random access of stored data and accommodate multiple users of the same system. Hard disc storage systems would allow for computers to impact more potential users (Hahn, 1996).

While hardware structures were changing in this period, the communications infrastructure they ran on was also being transformed. The establishment of Tymnet and Telenet in 1975 allowed computers to run across broadband networks. These developments provided for faster and more reliable access to data stored on computers. This would link computers into the national telecommunications framework, and make it possible for users to remotely tap into the information stored in distant databases (Perry, 1992).

OCLC

Libraries quickly saw the potential that enhanced computer capabilities would have in expanding the scope of cooperative endeavors. Computers were first applied to cooperative cataloging in trying to eliminate the problems associated with duplicate work. Many libraries were paying up to $60 per title to provide original cataloging service for every item they received (Mason, 1998). Fred Kilgour, when addressing this problem in Ohio, set up the Ohio College Library Center (OCLC) in 1967. Unlike other consortia arrangements of the time, Kilgour saw new computer technology as playing a central role in the cooperation he envisioned. Marilyn Mason talks about the founding ideals of OCLC:

> Kilgour believed that the solution to duplication was a shared effort that could be facilitated by information storage and retrieval systems that were becoming small enough to handle the load. He believed that instead of waiting for the top-down efforts of the Library of Congress, which were often slow and cumbersome, libraries could function as a single unit held together by wire and electronic pulses. He believed that a title could be cataloged once, by a library in Texas or Massachusetts, and that the efforts of that library could be shared with other libraries. (Mason, 1998)

The online OCLC database of cataloging records was established in 1971. This central electronic depository of cataloging records would dramatically increase access to information and reduce technical processing costs for libraries.

Starting with only 54 Ohio libraries, the expansion and success of OCLC was spectacular. Within a decade OCLC would grow to include 2,300 libraries and over 5 million records in the bibliographic system. In the late 1990s, OCLC would include 24,000 libraries and over 38 million records in its database. OCLC proved to be the largest and most sustained cooperative effort in library history. The OCLC database integrated cooperative cataloging into the technical service function of almost every library (Mason, 1998).

The demonstrated success of OCLC encouraged other projects to be built around automated systems. Existing and new consortia began to use computers as the principal architecture for their cooperation. In the 1980s and 1990s a new period of economic retrenchment made efficient cooperation through online systems an attractive option. The rising costs of materials and reduced budgets created an environment for libraries to seek electronically-based cooperative solutions in an effort to enhance services and provide more access (Alexander, 1999).

Electronic Reference and More Technological Change

The emergence of electronic reference tools and services began to influence the shape of cooperation. From the 1960s to the 1980s vast numbers of traditional print bibliographic tools were automated and became databases. Libraries began tapping into fee-based "databanks" like DIALOG, ORBIT, BRS, and Lexis-Nexis to retrieve bibliographic resources for users. Online reference was emerging as distinct from the print based reference desk. In the mainframe computer environment of the day, all of this activity was tightly controlled by the costs of access and the expertise of the reference librarian. Despite the built-in protocols of using such systems, both the librarian and the user were becoming increasingly aware of resources existing outside of their libraries (Straw, 2001).

Library control of online reference was shaken by the appearance of microcomputers in the early 1980s. IBM released the first microcomputer, using the MSDOS operating system, in 1981. Others soon followed and very quickly personal computing was opened up to the general public (Lenck, 1991). These personal computers were made more powerful by the emergence of a new networking technology in the 1990s. This technology linked computers together in a vast super network known as the Internet. The Internet had its origins in the linking of a number of government, university, and corporate computers in the late 1960s. More networks became active with the development of a Standard Internet Protocol in 1982, which allowed for communication between networks using different interfaces. By the mid 1990s, this IP standard would allow for the linking of tens of thousands of different networks around the world (Cere and Leiner, 1997).

Internet technology would get a further jolt by the emergence of the World Wide Web (WWW). The WWW is a hyper-linked, multimedia interface that can be used for retrieving information from the open Internet. The development of web browsers in the early 1990s made this an attractive and practical option for searching the Internet. After 1995 the WWW exploded on the scene and it currently is the most popular means for getting information from the Internet (Abbate, 1999).

The migration of personal computers and the WWW to libraries transformed the provision of reference services. Electronic searching is end-user driven with users able to access a world of information without intervention. More users can now tap into collections and services from libraries around the world creating a demand for information that is not held in local library collections. Clearly reference services today are less about finding things in a particular library, and more about connecting users to information anywhere.

Libraries have taken advantage of Internet technology to mount platforms and gateways to display locally important information. WWW interfaces are now used to access catalogs, reference databases, and general library services. Such platforms are also used to virtually extend the reference desk through the provision of e-mail and real time chat services (Stover, 2000). The demand and expense of such services have provided a strong motivation for cooperation in recent years. Banding together to purchase and provide access to electronic services is certainly a major concern of many contemporary consortia arrangements. The increased importance of access and technology is noted by William Potter:

> While the chief reason for academic libraries to form consortia has been to share existing resources, a new trend is becoming evident or at least more pronounced. Libraries are forming alliances for the purpose of identifying and addressing common needs arising from the developments in information technology, especially the

growing importance of the Internet and the World Wide Web. (Potter, 1997)

Combinations of libraries are now buying and providing access to databases, and making their reference expertise available to each other. Library cooperation in an electronic environment is clearly impacting the transformation of contemporary reference services.

With so much information for the taking, users are less focused on what any particular library might have in its collection. Libraries must be prepared to educate users about information wherever it may be found. In a world of cooperation and universal access, libraries must think about making users intelligent consumers of information. Librarians will have to think beyond there libraries and see their institutions as dynamic platforms that can link users to information anywhere. Helping users ask thoughtful questions, evaluate sources, and understand information structures will define the role of libraries in the future (Stover, 2000).

CONCLUSION

The idea of cooperation is strongly rooted in the library profession. The prevalence of library cooperation today is clearly the product of historical developments. Communication, transportation, and economic necessity have all impacted the shape cooperation has taken over the years. The technological change of the past 30 years has accelerated the pace of cooperation. With the barriers between libraries falling, libraries can no longer focus on their own collections. In the coming years, libraries will have to be prepared to help users retrieve and evaluate information wherever it is found.

REFERENCES

Abbate, Janet (1999), *Inventing the Internet*. Cambridge, MA: MIT Press.

Alexander, Adrian M. (1999), "Toward the Perfection of Work: Library Consortia in the Digital Age," *Journal of Library Administration* 28 (2), 1-14.

Ambrose, Lodilla (1890), "The Use of Books in One Library by the Readers in Another," *Library Journal* 15 (March), 68.

Belden, Charles F.D. (1921), "The Public Libraries and the Special Libraries," *Special Libraries* 12 (September-October), 180-181.

Bierbaum, Esther G. (1993), *Special Libraries in Action: Cases and Crises*. Englewood, Colo: Libraries Unlimited.

Bush, Vannevar (1945), "As We May Think," *Atlantic Monthly* 176 (1), 101-108.

Cere, Vinton G. and Leiner, Barry M (1997), "The Evolution of the Internet as a Global Information System," *International Information & Library Review* 29 (June), 129-151.

Fischer, Claude S. (1992), *America Calling: A Social History of the Telephone to 1940.* Berkeley, CA: University of California Press.

Fuller, Wayne E. (1972), *The American Mail: Enlarger of the Common Life.* Chicago, Ill: University of Chicago Press.

Green, Samuel S. (1876), "The Lending of Books to One Another by Libraries," *Library Journal* 1 (September), 15-16.

Hahn, Trudi B. (1996), "Pioneers of the Online Age," *Information Processing & Management* 32 (1), 33-48.

Kraus, Joe W. (1975), "Prologue to Library Cooperation," *Library Trends* 24 (October), 169-181.

Larned, Josephus N. (1897), "The Organization of Cooperative Work Among Public Libraries," *Transactions and Proceedings of the 2nd International Library Conference held in London, July 13-16, 1897.* New York: Houghton Mifflin.

Lenck, F. (1991), "History of the PC," *Computing Now* 9 (5), 12-15, 37.

Mason, Marilyn G. (1998), "Reference Revolutions," *Journal of Library Administration* 25 (2/3), 55-63.

Neufeld, Lynne M. and Cornog, Martha (1986), "Database History: From Dinosaurs to Compact Discs," *Journal of the American Society for Information Science* 37 (4), 183-190.

Patrick, Ruth J. (1972), *Guidelines for Library Cooperation.* System Development Cooperation.

Perry, Edwin (1992), "Historical Development of Computer Assisted Literature Searching and Its Effects on Librarians and Their Clients," *Library Software Review* 11 (March-April), 18-24.

Potter, William G. (1997), "Recent Trends in Statewide Academic Library Consortia," *Library Trends* 45 (Winter), 417-418.

Stover, John F. (1997), *American Railroads.* Chicago Ill: University of Chicago Press.

Stover, Mark (2000), "Reference Librarians and the Internet: A Qualitative Study," *Reference Services Review* 28 (1), 39-46.

Straw, Joseph E. (2001), "From Magicians to Teachers: The Development of Electronic Reference in Libraries: 1930-1970," *The Reference Librarian* 74, 1-12.

Symposium of Library Coordination and Inter-Library Loans (1910), *Library Journal* 35 (March), 101-102.

Stuart-Stubbs, Basil (1975), "An Historical Look at Resource Sharing," *Library Trends* 23 (April), 649-664.

Weber, David C. (1976), "A Century of Cooperative Programs Among Academic Libraries," *College & Research Libraries* 37 (May), 205-221.

Index

Active listening skills, 59
Agreements (consortial), 269-270
American Association of School
    Librarians, 86
American Library Association, 6-7,12,
    18-19,59-60,66
Androgyny theory (Knowles, M.),
    76-78
Antagonism alleviation, 135
Assistance acquisition, 46-49
Association for Educational
    Communications and
    Technology, 86
Association of College and Research
    Libraries, 66,86-87,125,
    141-142,194,197-200,220-221
Association of Research Libraries,
    146-147,207-208,221,228

Backhus, S.H., 2,193-202
Behavior-related competencies, 59-60
Berry, T.U., 2,145-155
Blending (resources), 119-130. *See
    also* Multi-faceted reference
    departments
Bloom, B.S., 75-77
Branch library contexts, 251-262. *See
    also* Combined service
    perspectives
Brooklyn College, 86,93-94
Bullian, J., 2,219-236
Burnout, 52-54
Burton, M., 2,71-81
Buxton, K.A., 2,251-262

Canned responses, 188-189
Case studies. *See also under individual
    topics*
of collection development aspects,
    145-155,228-234
of combined service perspectives,
    251-262
of customized library creation,
    237-250
of e-mail reference service, 183-191
of institution-specific programs. *See
    also under specific
    institutions*
    at Arizona State University,
        237-250
    at Brooklyn College, 86,93-94
    at Colorado College, 36-39
    Cooperative Library Project,
        86,93-94
    at Georgia State University,
        83-96
    at Hillsborough Community
        College, 231-233
    at Michigan State University,
        183-191
    at Missouri State University,
        203-218
    at Oregon State University,
        97-118
    at Pacific Northwest National
        Laboratory (Hanford
        Technical Library), 251-262
    at St. Charles Community
        College, 175-182
    at University of California
        (Davis), 85